Optimum Health

Making Conscious Choices

Andrea Switzer

with

Bob Switzer

Darcie,
I wish you the
greatest success on your
journey to achieving a
perpetual state of health,
happiness, and vitality!

ASwitzer

Optimum Health: Making Conscious

Printed by Createspace, North Charleston, SC, USA

Library of Congress Cataloguing-in-Publication Data

Switzer, Andrea; Switzer, Bob

Optimum Health: Making Conscious Choices

ISBN 13: 978-1494963408

ISBN 10: 149496340X

Alternative Health, Health & Fitness, Spirituality, Personal Growth

Disclaimer Statement

The suggestions given in this book are to help the reader make their own better, more conscious choices about behavior, lifestyle, modalities and professional medical support that suits their unique needs. Not all of the information, statements, advice, opinions, or suggestions contained in this book have been evaluated by the FDA or other health review authorities in other jurisdictions, and therefore should not be relied upon to diagnose, treat, cure, or prevent any condition, disease, illness or injury. This book is for informational purposes only. The authors, editor and publisher of this book do not provide medical advice or prescribe the use of any techniques for physical, emotional, mental or medical problems. The publisher, editor and authors do not make any claim as to the accuracy or appropriateness of any course of action described.

The intent of the authors is to only offer information of a general nature to help the reader in their quest for good health. In the event you use any of the information in this book for yourself, the authors, editor and the publisher assume no responsibility or liability for the use of any information or material in this book, or your actions or outcomes.

The authors and publisher are not affiliated with, do not endorse, and assume no responsibility for any individuals, entities or groups who claim to be manufacturing or marketing products or services referred to in this book, or who otherwise claim to be acting in accordance with any of the information or philosophies set forth herein.

The names of the storytellers have been changed for privacy and these contributors have signed a release giving the authors and publisher permission to use their stories. Many of these interviews also appear in Bob Switzer's book, Every Illness Has a Spiritual Solution.

This book is a reflection of the authors' own fitness, health and spiritual understandings and is not intended to speak for any spiritual path, teacher, or religion.

This book is written in Andrea Switzer's voice.

To the hundreds of students and clients I have worked with over the years, and to my countless course instructors, friends and family members, thank you for all you have taught me.

Table of Contents

Chapter 1   Making Conscious Choices   9

Chapter 2   Choose Your Foods Wisely   19

Chapter 3   Avoid Poisons in Your Environment   43

Chapter 4   Outgrow Emotional Toxins   63

Chapter 5   What You Believe, You Can Achieve   85

Chapter 6   Create Your Life Anew – Positively   107

Chapter 7   Developing Your Inner Guidance:

             Making Choices from Your Highest Perspective   123

Chapter 8   Fitness – Key to Optimum Health   135

Final Thoughts   155

Appendix   157

About the Author   159

1

Making Conscious Choices

We are a state of consciousness. Everyone and everything in our personal and universal world has an effect upon us. We want to become aware of what these effects are. Then we can sort through them, nurturing the good ones and discarding the bad.

Harold Klemp, Spiritual Wisdom on Health and Healing

I believe life is about balance, a balance of the right foods for you, the right exercise for your particular body and more. This "more" is being aware of environmental toxins, maintaining emotional balance, being conscious of how our attitudes, thoughts and beliefs shape our life, and finding a personal spiritual harmony of being, possibly even finding your life's purpose along the way.

Taken together, these elements have formed my approach to helping hundreds of clients achieve their goals in one-on-one training, group training, and small and large classes. It's really about making better, more conscious choices.

Human beings are bodies, minds and spirits. Health necessarily involves all of those components, and any program intended to improve health must address all of them.

Andrew Weil, MD

In the following pages, I'd like to share with you how your health is determined by the personal world you have created which has been shaped by the conscious and unconscious choices you have made up this point in your life. So after over 20 years of helping people work toward achieving optimum health I felt it was time to put what I have learned down in writing for my clients and students today and for anyone that wants to attain a new level of health and enthusiasm in life. My goal is to help you see how you can create a better, healthier YOU by making more conscious choices in all areas of your life – a body-mind-soul approach.

Let me introduce you to Jill.

Jill's Story

I became Jill's personal trainer two years after her accident and subsequent embarkation on a spiritual journey of awakening. Twenty-four months earlier she had regained consciousness in the crumpled body of a small commercial aircraft embedded in the side of a mountain on Vancouver Island. Here is what she told me:

...On January 21, 2006, my husband and I were enjoying a couple's massage during a romantic getaway and five hours later we were experiencing fifteen terrifying minutes of uncertainty as to whether we would live or die. The single engine plane suddenly lost all its power and the fate and destiny of all eight passengers on board was about to change forever. Flashing before me was my life... what had I done? What and who would I miss? More importantly, what was the meaning of those unfamiliar blue eyes that superimposed themselves over my husband's eyes minutes before we crashed? I somehow had a knowingness that I would survive and yet a feeling that Terry, my husband wouldn't.

I knew the moment we crashed there must be a much bigger reason for my surviving.

My story appears to be about the miraculous rescue, my survival, and of the trauma of losing Terry and my 'princess' life as I knew it. But, buried deep beneath the many layers of truth, the real 'soul' story emerges... which is of my spiritual transformation towards a life that I had thought was possible but had no idea how to get there. All of which had nothing to do with my material world that I had aspired to for most of my life. The spiritual path that I had been catapulted onto was certainly uplifting, unfamiliar and yet fascinating to me. I was 47, widowed and had a clean slate to begin my life over again. Undaunted by the magnitude of this tragedy, I took the road of uncertainty over despair. My long journey from recovery first began with eleven operations required to put humpty dumpty back together again. In fact, however, it was the emotional body that needed the most healing and where the reason for this accident began to unfold very clearly for me.

My journey inward in search of answers began by learning to meditate. Only because of the lengthy recovery time required was I able to see how perfect everything was - divinely inspired if you will. I needed that time to listen to what my soul had been trying all my life to get me to hear and see. My busy mind and Type A personality was not accustomed to slowing down, nor was I open to listening with my heart instead of my head. However, I soon learned that in the quiet state of mind... was where soul really spoke to me. During at least eighteen months of the total four years it took for my physical healing time, I was in this altered state of consciousness in which everything around me was coming from a state of LOVE. This state was so unusual and unfamiliar to me, particularity given the nature of this tragedy, that this time I knew I had to listen.

My fears had nothing to do with crashing in an airplane, but rather a much bigger picture that involved a lot of my own limiting beliefs about everything: men, position, trust, and of course my own self-worth.

As I peeled away the layers of some very deep-seated emotions like anger, resentment, and disappointment, I discovered that many of my beliefs that were valid and true for me before the accident were now on the table for questioning. I very much felt the 'disconnect' between my old thoughts and my new feelings.

I could see that some of these old behaviours, resulting from my subconscious limiting beliefs did not serve me anymore. The accident acted as a catalyst to allow me to see my truth and to take responsibility for my life. And when I changed how I perceived things, the things I perceived changed. For example, my body would heal and function optimally if I let go of the points of view that caused all my discomfort in the first place. When my anger and frustration diminished, my bowel irritability improved. And once I let go of carrying the weight of the world on my shoulders, my neck, back and shoulders stopped aching. Only when I perceived the accident as a gift did my body start to function with more ease.

Because of this heightened awareness, I also became aware of my dreams that were also leading me to my truth. Coincidentally and synchronisticly, all the right people including Andrea, places and things were simply lining up for me, to not only heal but more importantly to help me realize that I was meant to survive this accident, despite great odds, because there was something 'more' and 'bigger' for me to still do and or be.

My near death experience in the plane was when my soul was contemplating whether I should/could transition now OR, did I still have some unfinished business with regards to the contract that I had written before I even incarnated into this body. Having found the owner of "those eyes" in a new relationship, God had shown me how to gently open my heart again to love. My dreams gently suggested I start to look at all the events in my life, from childhood on, that led up to the accident. There are no accidents and there are no exceptions. So, given that Universal truth, I had to find a way to make sense of it all. After all, bad things don't happen to good people!

Before the crash I led with my brain, but this accident was helping me realize, in order to be happy and find true peace and harmony I needed to lead with my heart.

All my life, God has been whispering and nudging me along towards my true purpose... only I never listened. My lengthy recovery allowed me time to connect all the dots, as I examined every inch of my life. In doing so, I discovered many limiting beliefs about myself that were not going to serve me any longer in my expanded awareness of who I really was. I also discovered my 'shadow' self, the parts of my personality that I hadn't wanted to admit to, but in fact were true. When I faced my controlled and bullied childhood I learned to forgive my transgressors, for whom I had held so much silent anger inside of me, and to forgive them for all they had done to me. In fact, I also learned to forgive myself for allowing it to fester in my later years. Up until the accident, I had suffered in angry silence. I never spoke up and I didn't think I had anything important to say.

I also made the connections between the parts of my body that were injured and the parts afterwards that continued to not be in balance as to what I was still holding onto. My emotional body was speaking the loudest. When I didn't let go of my anger, I had trouble digesting my food and was constipated a lot, despite my now more active schedule and healthy eating. I felt out of balance in my lower chakras (energy centers) *which I was now able to see when I meditated. Once I could make those connections, I worked on that particular issue that related to that chakra.*

Our reactions to life-altering events are what make us either victims or victors in life. There are no accidents and there are no exceptions.

Through the excavation of all my stuff, I discovered that addictions and limiting beliefs are carried in the cellular memory in our DNA. This is why on a subconscious level we continue to attract the same types of people and situations into our lives – unless we are willing to look at these limiting beliefs about ourselves and take the necessary steps to change those beliefs. Until I was willing to look inside and change my limiting and negative beliefs, I would stay stuck in circumstances that would play out not only in this lifetime, but possibly every lifetime still to come.

Having the courage to change our perspectives and our limiting beliefs is not easy, but is each soul's journey – and it is worth it. It is a process and a journey all at the same time.

Each step of the way of recovery beautifully laid out for me some karmic lessons I needed to learn and address in this lifetime.

Challenging everything I once knew and believed, faith... a now knowingness of not only who I am as personality, but that we are simply souls having a human experience on Earth, and not a human having the occasional soulful experience. The other side is simply filled with unconditional love, acceptance, joy, peace, happiness and creativity. My new found faith allowed me to take the unfamiliar steps towards my authentic self and thus allowing me peace and freedom from this tragedy and more. I mostly heard... love more and simplify my life. Love and forgive myself and others for exactly who they are. It took a life-threatening event and near death experience to see this truth... I call my "plane" truth.

Jill was a wonderful client to work with on so many levels. She was taking responsibility for her circumstances and was willing to grow and uncover more about herself. She was willing to do what it takes to regain her health working on so many levels – physical, emotional, mental and spiritual – to gain a new total harmony of being.

∞

A Body-Mind-Soul Guide

This book serves as my guide for clients today, completed after many years of service to others, personal research into what I have found to work and attending numerous leading-edge educational fitness and health conferences. This book is also a synthesis of information from anatomy, physiology, kinesiology, nutrition, aromatherapy, reflexology and massage and comes about through practical application, extensive research, sharing and collaboration with other experts, and regular training programs.

These pages also reflect several years of spiritual study which has brought me new levels of awareness, creativity and the ability to make better choices in my life. Many of these personal awakenings have changed my view-point on health and fitness – taken me to a higher perspective so-to-speak – and so in the following pages through more stories, and my personal observations I'd also like to share some of these new realizations with you, as I have discovered they have a profound influence on our health.

Health is a state of complete harmony of the body, mind and spirit.

When one is free from physical disabilities and mental distractions,

the gates of the soul open.

B.K.S. Iyengar, founder of Iyengar Yoga

Making Conscious Choices

Making the right choices in our life takes a conscious effort. It means taking the time to distinguish between actions that contribute to our welfare and health and those that don't. It also means being able to discriminate between what will be best for our spiritual advancement or what would be wasting our time. It even comes down to deciding when to speak and when not to. In short, it means making conscious choices in all situations.

This involves getting to know yourself better. It means recognizing your weaknesses first, then deciding that you want to make better choices. Some of the choices I outline in the pages that follow are easy substitutions. Others may be a challenge for you. But I ask you to keep an open mind and if there is something I say that is not in harmony with your current beliefs, abilities or experience, just leave it and focus on the rest. Rome was not built in a day!

When you decide to make changes to improve your life, you will find that Spirit will also begin to support your good intentions. Don't be surprised if you see messages in your dreams more clearly or that your intuition gets stronger. This new level of attunement with your inner being, Soul, can manifest as a new knowingness and can be a big help in supporting the changes you feel can lead to a healthier you.

What you make out of life is up to you. You have free will. I believe we have been given all the skills, talents and tools we need to solve our challenges. Creativity is a key tool and includes going within through contemplation, meditation, prayer, quiet time and introspective activities such as yoga, running or walking. Imagination, visualization, asking for help, listening and being open to answers in whatever form they come, are an important part of the creative discovery process which is discussed in-depth in a coming chapter.

My wish is that you can benefit from all that I have learned from a holistic point-of-view (body, emotions, mind and soul) so that you can enrich your life in finding optimum health through making more conscious choices.

Let's start with foods that harm the body and foods that support good health.

Health is normal. The human body is a self-repairing, self-defending, self-healing marvel. Disease is relatively difficult to induce, considering the body's powerful immune system. However, this complicated and delicate machinery can be damaged if fed the wrong fuel during the formative years.

Healthy living with nutritional excellence throughout life can slow the decline of aging. It can prevent the years and years of suffering in ill health that is so common today as people get older and become dependent on medical treatments, drugs, and surgery. Nutritional excellence is the only real fountain of youth.

Joel Fuhrman, Disease-Proof Your Child: Feeding Kids Right

2

Choose Your Foods Wisely

If you want to live free of cancer, heart disease and diabetes for your entire life, that power is in your hands (and your knife and fork) but, sadly, medical schools, hospitals and government health care agencies continue to treat nutrition as if it only plays a minor role in health. And no wonder: the standard Western diet, along with its trendy "low fat" and "low carb" cousins is actually the cause, not the cure of what ails us.

T. Colin Campbell, PhD,

Whole: Rethinking the Science of Nutrition

Suzanne's Story

*U*p until a couple of years ago Suzanne had been on what she called a sugar roller coaster ride for thirty-five years. She had been moving in and out of good health due to her addiction to sugar. She told me, "I had inflamed sinuses and yeast infections throughout my body. When I ate excessive amounts of sugar, I also had bad headaches and an overall feeling of lethargy combined with bouts of depression."

Suzanne explained, "Early on I had seen my medical doctor and she had first diagnosed my condition as low blood sugar and then later she confirmed that it was Candida Yeast. My doctor recommended I go off all foods with sugar including bread. Honey and fruit were okay in moderation. But I was addicted to sugar. I'd go off these harmful foods, then I'd start cheating and have just a little, and then the addiction for sugar would grow again.

"I lived like this for years. Then a couple of years ago I had an attack. I had eaten some chocolate bars and not soon after, my brain felt like it was on fire. It really scared me! It was the final straw after years of ups and downs on and off sugar and the terrible symptoms that would accompany my cheating. I realized I could do permanent damage – something really dangerous – so feeling my brain on fire was finally enough to get my attention to quit completely. I've now been sugar free for two years.

Another Issue to Deal With

"Recently I went in to see my Naturopathic Doctor to check my metal toxicity levels and the results were the best I've ever had. But then the doctor started asking me other questions. She inquired about a few things like, 'Do you eat out of a microwave?' My answers were negative but she revealed that my body was not absorbing vitamins and minerals and this would cause problems down the road. She told me that she suspected gluten intolerance and explained that the gluten could be causing an allergic reaction in my intestines. They would be inflamed as a result and then not be able to absorb the nutrients.

"I immediately accepted the gluten-free diet and I later found out even a crumb will weaken me, causing a severe reaction that would take several weeks to recover from; I discovered there was a bit of wheat in mixed nuts! Lately I've eliminated all processed foods and I'm eating a far healthier whole food diet. I even dine out less now and I feel great, happy, I have energy and I'm feeling like I'm loving life – not focussed on food.

A Larger Shift

"I had had many gentle nudges that I ignored, but when I was in the doctor's office, it all came into focus for me. This food shift has ushered in a new energy for me. I'm feeling much kinder and gentler these days and I've started reading a powerful series of books, The Ringing Cedars Series by Vladimir Megre, which talk about being more loving to Earth and promoting a whole new way of being. So this shift is on many levels and the departure from gluten has been a catalyst for a larger repositioning involving many changes. I've even decided to let go of my old first name which no longer fits me; I was called Suzie and I've now softened it to Suzanne, my legal name.

"This whole change has also brought into focus for me how important every thought, feeling and action is and has moved me into a greater awareness of the present moment, and my impact on the world in every moment. It's shifted me toward being more loving and kind to everyone I meet and with whom I share my life.

"The process has made me realize how I need to purify myself on all levels, and to do this to be the most benefit to my planet, my world. I ask myself, 'How can I be better, more kind, more loving?'

"I'm looking for how I can open up a little more and impact life in a positive way."

∞

Life is a Moving Target

Like Suzanne, what you could eat in the past may be causing you issues today as you age and move along your life path. Certain foods are known to cause problems in many people (e.g. gluten) and other foods may only affect a select few (peanuts). And then there are foods that have not been proven to cause any problems but may be a problem for you. (I have a problem with red meat.) Don't discount any possibilities. Life is a moving target! As you grow older, many foods or food products may become incompatible with your system and therefore toxic in your body. This may start as a mild discomfort, progress to an irritation, and finally move to a very visible condition and outright pain. In other cases, there may be no direct signal at all, just a feeling of loss of energy, a malaise, or other subtle symptom that is not related to a particular action, product or food type. What I'm saying here is that you need to expect to make changes and that you may need to remove things from your sphere on a trial basis and monitor the effects. Let's start with a look at mass consumption foods.

Why Are We Such a Sick Society?

Despite the most advanced medical technology in the world, we are sicker than ever by nearly every measure. Two out of every three are overweight, cases of diabetes are exploding, especially in the younger population and about half are taking at least one prescription drug. (Obesity is the second most preventable cause of death; cigarette smoking is first.) Major medical operations have become routine, helping to drive health care costs to astronomical levels. Heart disease, cancer and stroke are leading causes of death, even though billions are spent each year to "battle" these very conditions. Many others are dealing with a host of other degenerative diseases.

The China Study, a 20-year study that began in 1983 and was conducted jointly by the Chinese Academy of Preventive Medicine,

Cornell University, and the University of Oxford examined mortality rates from 48 forms of Cancer and other chronic diseases. It concluded that counties in China with a high consumption of animal-based foods were more likely to have had higher death rates from "Western" diseases, while the opposite was true for counties that ate more plant foods. The study was conducted in those counties because they had genetically similar populations that tended, over generations, to live in the same way in the same place, and eat diets specific to those regions.

The conclusion: that most, if not all, of the degenerative diseases that afflict us can be controlled, or even reversed, by altering our present menu of animal-based and processed foods.

A Plant Strong Diet

Forks Over Knives is a recent video documentary that examined this thesis. Discoveries inspired by Doctors Campbell and Esselstyn, are examined and their years of groundbreaking studies presented. The documentary concluded that diseases like heart disease, type 2 diabetes, and even several forms of cancer, can almost always be prevented—and in many cases reversed—by adopting a whole-foods, plant-based diet. These doctors recommend a plant-rich diet, scaling way back or eliminating altogether foods such as red meat, poultry, fish, and dairy products. Despite the profound implications of their findings, their work has remained relatively unknown to the public.

Results are reported as rapid and dramatic when a switch is made. Depending on your health, you may wish to do your own three or four week test.

Heart Disease Findings

Dr. Dwight Lundell, a heart surgeon with 25 years experience, having performed over 5,000 open-heart surgeries, says inflammation is the primary cause of heart disease. He asks, "What are the biggest culprits of chronic inflammation? Quite simply, they are the overload

23

of simple, highly processed carbohydrates (sugar, flour and all the products made from them) and the excess consumption of omega-6 vegetable oils like soybean, corn and sunflower that are found in many processed foods."

Maintaining Good Health

There are certain foods that could almost be called miracle foods, and they are all around us. What I find so tragic in our Western culture is that we have easy access to high-quality foods yet we are avoiding them in favour of convenience foods, processed foods and junk. Today's research is pointing out to us that just by adding some value-packed foods to our diet we can stay incredibly healthy well into our later years.

The excuse seems to be a shortage of time, yet these whole fresh foods I'm referring to can be made ready to eat in the same time as prepared and processed foods. I'm talking about steaming vegetables and making a simple salad for example. Or simply adding a miracle fruit like blueberries or a vitamin rich vegetable such as broccoli to your diet as part of a meal or as a snack. As the unique being that you are you may not be able to tolerate in your diet what the masses can. You may need to augment your food choices with some highly nutritious foods if you are not already doing so. This is an easy place to make some new choices!

What is Hidden Hunger?

The effects of hidden hunger can impair individuals, sapping their energy, productivity and mental ability. Hidden hunger is caused by a chronic lack of essential vitamins and minerals. People often don't realize they are suffering from hidden hunger and this can have potentially devastating effects. Hidden hunger can result from an overreliance on processed foods including fast foods and not eating fresh fruits and vegetables.

For example, a lack of Vitamin A can impair the immune system and make children more vulnerable to diseases such as measles, diarrhea, and malaria. A fetus or infant that suffers from iodine deficiency may become mentally impaired. A lack of iron can cause anaemia in women and children and mental impairment in growing children. Women who do not have enough folic acid are more likely to become anaemic and to have children with neural tube birth defects.

Delaying a meal brings about symptoms most people call "hunger." These symptoms include abdominal cramping, weakness, and feeling ill -the same as during drug withdrawal. This is not hunger. Our dietary habits, especially eating animal-protein-rich foods three times a day, are so stressful to the detoxification system in our liver and kidneys that we start to get withdrawal, or detoxification symptoms the minute we aren't busy processing such food. Real hunger is not that uncomfortable.
Dr. Joel Fuhrman

Micronutrients

Micronutrients are now becoming better known as essential to good health. These nutrients are required by humans and other living things in small quantities throughout life to orchestrate a whole range of physiological functions, but which the organism itself cannot produce.

Micronutrients are needed only in minuscule amounts, yet can be considered miracle elements that enable the body to produce enzymes, hormones and other substances essential for proper growth and development. As tiny as the amounts are, however, the consequences of their absence are severe. Iodine, Vitamin A and iron are most important in terms of our health. **Other micronutrients** include chromium, copper, manganese, selenium, zinc and molybdenum.

Dr. Joel Fuhrman is a big proponent of micronutrients and recommends the following six "super foods" to be included in a healthy diet:

> salad greens,
>
> onions,
>
> mushrooms,
>
> beans,
>
> berries,
>
> and seeds.

Others say these foods are also cancer inhibiting foods. Dr. Fuhrman's suggestion is to eat a salad every day with these ingredients for optimum health. What could be simpler!

Supplements

A detailed discussion on supplements is beyond the scope of this book, BUT, know that supplements alone cannot offer optimal protection against disease, and you cannot make an unhealthy diet into a healthy one by consuming supplements. There is also a growing body of evidence that is saying many supplements are overrated in their effectiveness and may even contain harmful ingredients as T. Colin Campbell states:

> *...the limited efficacy of supplements reflects the limited science that created them: nutrients outside of their natural food context do little good and sometimes do considerable harm.*

T. Colin Campbell, PhD, Whole, Rethinking the Science of Nutrition and Coauthor of the China Study

He also says:

The 'magic bullet' love affair of supplementation lets us believe we're 'off the hook' when it comes to eating right. Why eat your vegetables when you can binge on hot dogs and ice cream and, if you get in trouble, make it all better with a pill.

Vitamin E

Vitamin E is another essential for good health. Processed foods, alcohol, tobacco, and smog increase your need for Vitamin E. Fatigue, stress and pollution can deplete it. Heat, oxygen, freezing and chlorine destroys Vitamin E.

Foods that are rich in Vitamin E include seeds, nuts, soy beans, brown rice, oats, fresh wheat germ and free range eggs. Also beneficial are dark green leafy vegetables, Brussels sprouts and broccoli.

Antioxidants

Antioxidants (anti-oxygen) are your first line of defence against free radicals. Free radicals are a normal part of metabolism and play a vital role in many biochemical processes, but they must be kept under control. To counteract these radical oxidants, the brain needs an ample supply of antioxidants. Basically, antioxidants are molecules that free radicals find more attractive than our body's cellular components.

Antioxidants can be found in micronutrients obtained from food. There are many different kinds of micronutrients that function as antioxidants to neutralize, or quench, free radicals. Each works in a unique manner and has a particular area of focus, but they also complement each other in an extraordinary synergy that effectively controls free radicals.

United States Department of Agriculture (USDA) nutritionists examined more than 100 different kinds of fruits, vegetables, nuts, spices, cereals and other foods for their antioxidant content. The results weren't altogether surprising: fruits, vegetables and beans claimed all the spots.

Here are the USDA top 20 antioxidant foods:

1. Small red bean (dried),
2. Wild blueberry,
3. Red kidney bean (dried)
4. Pinto bean,
5. Blueberry (cultivated),
6. Cranberry,
7. Artichoke (cooked hearts),
8. Blackberry,
9. Prune,
10. Raspberry,
11. Strawberry,
12. Red delicious apple,
13. Granny Smith apple,
14. Pecan,
15. Sweet cherry,
16. Black plum,
17. Russet potato,
18. Black bean (dried),
19. Plum,
20. Gala apple.

The number one antioxidant-rich food, small red beans (dried), at the top of the list are sometimes called a Mexican red bean, but they are actually only grown in Alberta, Washington and Idaho.

A Source of Potential Health Problems

In today's world of chemical agriculture, too many fertilizers herbicides and insecticides can play mayhem with our bodies allowing free radicals to attack us.

Today's large-scale farming methods and many genetically modified foods necessitate farmers use fertilizers, insecticides and herbicides to produce crop yields at market prices. It's a highly competitive business. Unfortunately, these chemicals end up in our food. Of course "everyone" is eating these foods but as I previously mentioned, your personal tolerance to these unwanted chemical residues may be lower than the average person's ability to resist their effects.

Here are some foods to monitor for your own ability to assimilate and remain in good health, or to buy organic:

apples,
celery,
strawberries,
peaches,
spinach,
nectarines (imported),
grapes (imported),
sweet bell peppers,
potatoes,
blueberries,
lettuce,
kale,
collard greens,
apricots,
green beans,
cherries.

The Issue with Vegetable Oils

Did you know that vegetable oil is not made with vegetables? It's manufactured from combinations of corn oil, soybean oil, canola oil, safflower oil, and/or cottonseed oil, which can be harmful to your health. It usually contains trans-fat and oxidized mutated fats as a result of the refining process; free radicals formed during the refining of vegetable oils create these mutated fats which damage cell membranes & chromosomes, and create inflammation in the body. Another cause of inflammation is that these oils are mostly made up of inflammatory omega-6 fats, while having very little anti-inflammatory omega-3 fats. The free radicals in vegetable oils also damage arteries, which can directly lead to a heart attack.

The more conscious choices of oil for cooking is organic coconut oil or organic virgin olive oil, and for your salads, organic virgin olive oil. The European brands are best as their legal definition of "virgin" is first pressing, while the usual North American definition of "virgin" allows numerous pressings.

Soy Products – Are They a Problem for You?

Numerous studies have found that food products containing soy can affect the health of some people. In North America soybeans are typically grown with pesticides and herbicides as most soy crops are genetically modified. If you are having health issues such as a thyroid disorder, kidney stones, and food allergies, as in all issues you are dealing with, I encourage you to do your own research on the Internet etc. (It's easy to simply type in to the search bar words like "soy issues, problems, symptoms etc.)

Obesogens, Hidden Causes of Weight Gain

"Obesogen" is a relatively new term that has emerged to describe a substance or food that contributes in some way to increased weight gain or obesity. An obesogen is a natural or synthetic chemical that is an endocrine-disruptor. Simply put, these chemicals disrupt the function of hormonal systems and metabolism, leading to weight gain. Obesogens enter our bodies different ways:

• Hormones given to animals;

• Plastics in food and drink packaging;

• Ingredients added to processed food; and

• Pesticides sprayed on produce.

Obesogens can cause damage because they mimic human hormones such as estrogen, they miss-program stem cells to be fat cells and they can possibly alter gene functions.

Where do you find them? The short answer: everywhere, particularly because high fructose corn syrup, which can be found in every kind of food, from sodas to yogurt to pretzels, is an obesogen. The ubiquitous, viscous sweet stuff makes your liver insulin resistant and tampers with leptin to increase your hunger, setting up a vicious cycle where you crave more food that is then more easily turned into fat.

Doctoroz.com (Doctor OZ's website for the Dr. OZ TV Show)

The Top Six Obesogens

High Fructose Corn Syrup is an ingredient in many packaged and processed foods. The main problem is that because it is so abundant and so cheap, it has found its way even into foods like pretzels and hamburger buns.

Animal and Fish Protein. In many animals, obesogens are stored in their fat. Be aware of some Atlantic and Farm-Raised fish which can have more pesticides in them and be artificially colored to look like wild salmon.

Tap Water. Because of the pesticides used in farming, those pesticides seep into the soil and the water table below. The best way to prevent these obesogens getting into your drinking water is to use a granular activated carbon (GAC) filter for your water purification.

Also check your municipal water supplier for their water quality report to see what's in your water.

Things around your house that contain obesogens. First is Bisphenol A or BPA a synthetic estrogen found in many plastics. This has been banned from baby bottles for years, but canned baby formula is lined inside the can with BPA. Also fatty and acidic foods that come in cans are lined with BPA, like tomato products and tuna. Experts recommend purchasing tuna in pouches that do not contain BPA and limiting the tomato products to those in jars or to do your own canning of tomato products. The other things to be conscious of are hard plastic water bottles with #7 in the triangle stamped on the bottom. Never microwave in containers made of plastic. BPA-free plastics contain triangles on the bottom with numbers 1, 2, 4, 5 and 6. Plastics with numbers 3 or 7 have no guarantee that they do not contain BPA.

Perfluorooctanoic acid or PFOA is another concern found in the home. It is a substance that makes things non-stick on pots, pans and cooking utensils. PFOA can impact your thyroid gland. One suggestion is to use wooden utensils for cooking because metal can scrape the coating which can end up in your food. PFOA is also found in microwave popcorn and pizza delivery boxes.

Also, be aware of **polyvinyl chloride or PVC** which release phthalates which lower testosterone and lowers metabolism so fat cannot be burned efficiently. These are found on vinyl shower curtains, especially liners. When taking a shower, combined with hot water, you are in a phthalate bath and inhaling this substance. Meat from the supermarket wrapped in see-through plastic wrap is loaded with PVC in the industrial/commercial strength, but home use wrap is not. I suggest going to a butcher who will wrap your meat in brown paper instead.

North American wheat is now coming under examination. According to Cardiac Specialist Doctor William Davis, author of *Wheat Belly*, it can now be a major contributor to weight gain and a large belly.

Just as the tobacco industry created and sustained its market with the addictive properties of cigarettes, so does wheat in the diet make for a helpless, hungry consumer. From the perspective of the seller of food products, wheat is a perfect processed food ingredient: The more you eat, the more you want. The situation for the food industry has been made even better by the glowing endorsements provided by the US government urging Americans to eat more 'Healthy' whole grains.

William Davis, MD, Wheat Belly

When my husband stopped eating wheat he dropped ten pounds and lost his belly. We substituted coconut flour bread, one hundred percent rye bread, and rice pasta and more recently I have been baking my own eight grain bread for the two of us. While travelling in South America and Europe, I have found that these local wheat food products do agree with my system.

Other areas to research that could be hidden contributors to weight gain are alcohol, hydrogenated oils (coconut oil and extra virgin olive oils are good alternatives), food additives and fast foods. So be aware of the things that can hinder your metabolism and hurt you and your family.

Food Additives, another Area of Concern

Used primarily to preserve shelf life and boost flavour, as well as to maintain colour, many synthetic additives have undergone inadequate, conflicting or inconclusive testing. While none of them have been definitively proven to be harmful, they haven't been proven to be safe, either; so being the unique being that you are, some additives may not be contributing to your good health.

A good website for doing your own research is *Center for Science in the Public Interest*. For the Center's complete list of additives and their accompanying safety rating visit the food safety section of its website.

The real message is that if you are trying to improve your health, try to eliminate foods with additives from your diet, even if for a test period and eat only fresh fruits, vegetables and meats. Monitor the results for a month of two, keeping a record of how you feel in your journal each day.

Gluten, a Hidden Cause of Health Issues

Many people today are suffering from issues that their doctors are unable to diagnose. These include migraine or headaches, joint pains or aches, brain fog, frequent bloating or gas, IBS, acid reflux, diarrhea or chronic constipation, depression or anxiety, ongoing fatigue and chronic eczema or acne. Dr. Oz (at doctoroz.com) says four or more symptoms indicate that gluten may be impacting your health. But even one symptom, if severe and chronic, like Suzanne experienced, can be a sign of gluten sensitivity. You may want to consult your doctor or easier yet, try going gluten-free for 2-4 weeks. Gluten free means eliminating wheat, rye and barley from your diet. Good substitutes include rice or quinoa pasta and rice flour or coconut flour bread as I have mentioned and added to my diet.

Are You Lactose Intolerant?

Those who are lactose intolerance or have a lactase deficiency cannot metabolize lactose properly; they lack *lactase*, an enzyme required in the digestive system to break down lactose. Lactose is a sugar that is found most notably in milk. Lactose intolerance is characterized by nausea, bloated stomach, abdominal pain, flatulence, diarrhea and cold sweats after consumption of food that contains lactose (milk, ice cream, cheese). The symptoms can range from mild discomfort to severe, depending on how much lactase one produces and the extent of their consumption of milk and other dairy products. I have also heard of people with skin conditions such as lumps under the skin that disappeared when they began avoiding dairy food products.

Your pH Balance

What you are eating could also be throwing off your body's pH balance into the acidic range. It is not healthy to be too acidic (nor too alkaline for that matter). pH represents the balance of positively charged (acid-forming) ions to negatively charged (alkaline forming) ions in your body. A low pH means you are too acidic. For optimum health your body should be slightly alkaline, however most North Americans are too acidic due to emotional and physical stress and the foods being consumed. This can cause toxic build-up, lack of absorption of important minerals and vitamins and free radical oxidation resulting in frequent colds and flu, weight gain, poor hair and skin and low bone density. More seriously, doctors have linked acidity with the proliferation of cancer cells. An alkaline pH discourages cancer development.

Key things to be aware of that cause acidity in the body include a strong reliance on processed foods, alcoholic beverages, sugars, hard and processed cheese, artificial sweeteners and red meat. Your local health food store can provide you with lots of suggestions for testing and balancing your pH levels.

If you have too much bad bacteria in your gut, it's going to extract calories from the foods you eat and store it as fat.
JJ Virgin, author of JJ Virgin's Sugar Impact Diet

Making Changes

You might be saying, what's next? How can I start making changes? There are a few simple things you can commit to, that require little will-power or sacrifice. Implement the common sense actions below recommended by a host of experts, and you are bound to improve your health and maintain it.

1. Keep fruits like apples and bananas out on your counter. You'll be more likely to eat them if you have to look at them every day!

2. Eat a salad every day for lunch or with every meal. Make it a rule. It doesn't matter what you are eating, just get a side salad. Skip the dressing if you can and just squeeze a little lemon juice and salt/pepper on top or balsamic vinegar and extra virgin olive oil.

3. Focus on adding nutrient dense foods, instead of subtracting unhealthy food from your diet. It is easier to add than subtract. Over time, you will get used to eating the leafy greens, and find it easier to cut back on your serving of processed foods.

4. Avoid refined sugars.

5. Drink lots of water.

Today, more than 95% of all chronic disease is caused by food choice, toxic (livestock) feed ingredients, nutritional deficiencies, and lack of physical exercise.

Mike Adams, The Health Ranger

Making Beneficial *Changes*

What food can you give up that is potentially harmful to you now or in the future?

Write down one thing that you can let go of that is no longer serving your best health interests - e.g. refined sugars, a food additive, hydrogenated oils, chemical sugar substitutes, wheat.

Letting Go of Certain Foods

My husband's personal journey is a good example of letting go of certain foods over time as he discovered one-by-one they made him feel ill or negatively affected him in some way. In his teens, he let go of chocolate. In his twenties he terminated refined sugars and all the confectionary foods and drinks he consumed. In his thirties, he had to drop coffee and alcohol and became vegetarian. A few years later, he added back into his diet fish and poultry. In his forties he added back in red meat after being diagnosed as borderline anaemic, revealed in a live blood cell analysis. He also let go of juices and started to only drink water. In his fifties, he had to let go of wheat due to bloating in his belly. He also discovered that he had a genuine sensitivity to MSG. He started to get a red flare above his lip if he ingested just a small amount of this substance. In recent years he's had to let go of eggs, snack foods with hydrogenated oil and garlic, and he can only tolerate milk if it is organic.

As I'm writing this book, we are now cutting back our meat consumption and emphasizing fresh organic vegetables and fruits, and fresh olive oil and coconut oil in our diets. We have also purchased a new water filter system that produces natural alkaline water.

My husband says that with all of the changes that he's had to make, he's still grateful for the many foods he can still enjoy, but he's still careful not to overindulge in any one particular food which could create an imbalance. The key for him is being open to what his body is telling him and making the changes, often with experimentation to be sure he was doing the right thing. These changes are the price of optimum health.

Review Your Diet

Review the following and rate yourself on how these could be affecting your health:

Substances: Wine, beer, alcohol, drinks containing caffeine and recreational substances will affect your journey at some point. Be prepared to make changes here! (Alcohol abuse doubles your risk of Alzheimer's.)

Drinks: Soda pop, coffee, tea, fruit juices, milk – many of these are exposed to pesticides and possibly herbicides and many carry levels of sugar which could be causing you problems.

Foods: Do you buy processed foods?

What ingredients/additives do these contain?

Foods around the store perimeter like meats, vegetables, fruit, and dairy tend to be better for us than processed foods but you may need to determine what exposure they have had to chemicals at source or in processing.

Processed meat products are loaded with ingredients that could be harmful to your unique constitution.

Don't overlook gluten and the obesogens previously mentioned.

Microwave: Do you microwave your food or beverages? There is controversy about what microwaving does to food and water. As the unique being that you are, this could be a source of problems for you.

My Diet at Present

Here is a snapshot of my food and beverages at present:

Key dietary influences: I make green smoothies and I use homemade almond or hemp milk, or store bought organic coconut beverage on my cereal (an organic home-made granola). I bake our own bread, made from eight grain cereal plus coconut and spelt flour that is wheat free. I eat lots of salads mostly at lunchtime and I eat chicken and fish but the portions are small. My husband and I are eating organic as much as possible, particularly the high risk fruits and vegetables.

My favorite snacks: fruit, nuts and home-made granola bars occasionally.

Foods I have left behind: wheat (North American), sugary products, deserts, most foods containing additives, preservatives and hydrogenated oils, and all fast foods.

Most noticeable beneficial addition: coconut oil – I use it on my skin as a moisturizer and sun screen (in addition to pure essential oil blends), and as a cooking oil. I also have a custom-made aromatherapy anti-wrinkle serum that I have made for myself.

My goal in writing this chapter has been to highlight several foods, food groups and additives that could be causing problems for you and give you some ideas where you can begin to easily make changes, taking charge of your health. As said before, you are unique and your sensitivities are as well. What others are able to eat can be causing you issues, so feel free to experiment and selectively add or subtract foods from your diet and monitor the way you feel a few weeks at a time.

Life expectancy would grow by leaps and bounds if green vegetables smelled as good as bacon.

Doug Larson, Newspaper Columnist

Making Conscious Choices - My Top Suggestions:

Current Choice	Issue	Conscious Choice
Food Sources		
Shopping the whole store	Processed	Shop the Perimeter
Processed Foods	Additives	Whole Foods
Factory Farms	GMO/Chemicals	Organic Farms/local
Meat-based Diet	Western Diseases	Plant Based Diet
Brand Name Honey	Pollen removed	Local Honey Farmer
Atlantic Salmon	Chemicals	Wild Salmon
Tap Water	Residues	Reverse Osmosis (R.O.)
Foods		
Sugar, Agave	Numerous	Honey, Maple Syrup
Artificial Sweeteners	Toxic	Honey, Maple Syrup
Wheat Bread (N. American)	Wheat Belly	100% Rye, Rice or Coconut
Pasta (wheat)	Wheat Belly	Rice or Quinoa Pasta
Vegetable Oils	Rancidity	Coconut or Olive Oil
Salad Dressing	Rancidity	Olive Oil & Vinegar
Margarine	Obesogen	Organic Butter
Hard Cheese	Acidic	Soft Cheese
Tuna	Mercury	Fresh Fish
Tinned Chicken	Corn starch	Fresh Chicken
Junk Foods	Toxic	Fresh Food Snacks
Peanuts	Toxic Mold	Mixed Nuts
Roasted Nuts	Rancidity	Salted or Plain Nuts

Juice	Ingredients	Home Made Juice
Soy Products	Chemicals	Organic Soy
Corn Syrup	Obesogen	Local Honey
Milk	Additives	Almond Beverage
Vitamins	Additives	Organic Salads & Fruit
Supplements	Additives	Nutritious Whole Foods

Packaging & Preparation

Frozen Foods	Obesogens	Fresh Foods/Salads
Tinned Tomatoes	Chemicals	Tomatoes in Glass Jars
Plastic Food Storage	Chemicals	Glass Food Storage
Water in plastic	Residues	R.O Filtered Water
Preservatives/MSG	Toxic	Natural/Organic Foods
Microwave Cooking	Nutrient Value	Steam or Stove Heat Foods
Non-stick Cookware	Chemicals	Steel/Glass Cookware

If you are going to eat foods made by people in white lab coats, you're going to end up seeing people in white lab coats.

Joe Cross, Fat, Sick & Nearly Dead: How Fruits and Vegetables Changed My Life

3

Avoid Poisons in Your Environment

Clinical ecology (is) a new branch of medicine aimed at helping people made sick by a failure to adapt to facets of our modern culture, polluted environment. Adverse reactions to processed foods and their chemical contaminants, and to indoor and outdoor air pollution with petrochemicals, are becoming more and more widespread and so far these reactions are being misdiagnosed by mainstream medical practitioners and so are not treated effectively.

Richard Mackarness, MD – Clinical Ecologist

Jessica's Story

*A*bout 9 years ago, Jessica told me she began to feel more and more tired, like her adrenals were tapped. She told me, "When I was under stress it was more pronounced, and following some immigration procedures that required vaccination for Measles, Mumps and Rubella, as well as a TB test I noticed a significant decline in my health. My body was very tired and a lot weaker."

Jessica's weakness persisted for several years, then things shifted for the worse. "About a year ago, I went through a period of high stress, studying late for several nights for an exam. At the same time, diarrhea started and got progressively worse, to the point where I was experiencing it around twelve times per day. My body was not absorbing anything and the added stress of starting a new job added to my toxic load. I lost twenty pounds in short order."

"I started doing research on-line for the possible causes of diarrhea and discovered the Specific Carbohydrate Diet. This is a diet high in carbohydrates that I began and it took the diarrhea down to about three times a day. Concurrently I'd been seeing my medical doctor who is also a Herbologist and she was busy ruling out all kinds of possible causes. She had heavy metals on her list of possibilities, but seemed to be looking in other areas. She recommended a colonoscopy, but the cost made me pause to consider whether this was the right course of action.

"My husband and I had been doing muscle testing on my condition across a wide range of options and we came up with a positive on heavy metals, so on the next visit, my intuition was so strong that I was insistent with my doctor that I have a heavy metals test. The test results showed that I had off-the-charts poisoning for mercury and lead!

Jessica told me, "My doctor started me on chelation therapy, however, the chelation pills gave me brain fog. I couldn't remember what I was doing and I'd put things where they didn't belong. I also had nausea and even threw up, and the diarrhea flared up again. I soon discovered that tests are only an indication of conditions, not conclusive. The chelation dosage was too much for my body and was making my predicament terrible, to the point that I was not functional - not able to work. In her notes about what helps, my medical doctor said that heavy metals collect in the bowels along with other places and that colonics were recommended as being very helpful. Well, I have been an enema pro for many years because my immune system has been less than robust, so as soon as I started doing enemas, my diarrhea settled down. The only time I got it again was after chelation therapy, when the metals had been pulled out of all the places my body had stashed it, and they collected in my bowels.

Turning the Corner

"When I started chelation, my brother-in-law an intuitive/spiritual healer, heard about my condition and offered to assist me. I accepted and he took a look at my test results. In his treatments he began pulling the metals out of my body which made me very ill from trying to process the metals to eliminate them, but this was when I began to turn the corner. During one of his treatments, he said to me, 'Why is it that I love your body more than you do?' His statement jarred me. In that moment I realized that I didn't love my body!

"At the time, I was so drained that I'd abandoned my spiritual practices and physical exercise. I now realize how critical these are to good health and balance. I began to write in my journal about the issue that was surfacing about not loving my body and I came to the conclusion that I have never felt good enough. So I began writing fantastic things regarding myself and one day a message came through: *God thinks you're good enough!* I cried for five minutes when I had that realization. This was so huge for me that I made signs and put them up around the house.

"I had also started up again doing my daily spiritual practices, a visualization where I imagine white light vibrating every cell in my body and aura. As well, I had renewed my daily prayers where I ask for inner guidance and then I thank God for what I've received."

When I asked Jessica about her level of involvement in her process of recovery, she replied, "All along I felt I'd been taking responsibility for my condition because I could see it was my karmic pattern: I knew I had to be very involved in the process which had led me to muscle testing and the help I received from my husband, brother-in-law and God.

Awakening to Self-limiting Beliefs

"When I turned the corner, it was really an awakening about self-limiting beliefs and it was my condition that helped me come to this realization – it was all the digging and soul-searching I was doing. My realization has helped me let go of the constant stress that was emanating from these deeply hidden feelings of not being good enough. In this journey, I've discovered that this feeling of a lack of self-worth was really a hidden fear, so I'm now better able to clearly identify what thoughts are mine as opposed to those that are negative.

"I'm now loving my body and knowing it is doing the very best it can given what I've put into it and the stresses I've created for it. And I'm loving it in spite of everything I had to go through."

Jessica shared another realization she has had: "Loving yourself gives you greater love for others," she told me. "It helps you have a greater understanding and then caring for others.

"Today, I feel I'm more loving, but it's just starting. The metals dull a lot of feeling in the brain and as I eliminate them I am freer to have more emotional sensitivity and perception. My mantras are burning up old karma - old patterns - these days and my visualization powers and concentration are now better as I get rid of the metals in my body. I could be a completely different person at the end of this process! As I move into who I am and who I'm going to be, I know I have to be aware of the old me when it emerges, and let it go. So I'm keeping up with my spiritual practices. I need to slow my processes down so I can let go of old thoughts, behaviors and actions as they come up."

Jessica has traced the source of her mercury poisoning to vaccinations and lead poisoning from living in close proximity to a major expressway and an airport for many years.

∞

Being Conscious of Change

An obvious place for taking responsibility for your health and well-being is in the physical environment. As you go through life, your body changes and so does your environmental setting. In all likelihood, what you could consume or tolerate in or on your body in your youth is going to change. This is a natural part of growing or aging. You need to accept this fact and know that you are going to have to make changes as you proceed if you want to stay in balance.

You are Unique

In addition, you need to appreciate that you are a unique being. What others can do or tolerate in and on their bodies may not be compatible with your body. You cannot judge yourself by what others can do. You have your own individual package of karma, genetic dispositions, emotions, sensitivities and preferences that attract you to certain environments, personal products, foods, work environments, residential settings etc. You are a one-of-a kind being and your tests and challenges in this life are also a custom package. These lessons are for your personal growth as Soul, so what works for everyone else may not suit you, and this includes what you eat, drink, what you do for exercise, work at, finances, and what you experience in your state of being. What is enjoyable to you may not be fun at all to somebody else. As such, your approach to life including your imbalances and disharmonies will also require a customized approach.

Key Questions to Ask

In examining your material world, this physical world, there are some key questions to ask yourself if you are seeking improved health.

Has anything changed in your relationships, house, home life, work, entertainment, vehicle, financial life and hobbies? Changes in your life may have brought new intolerances or toxic substances into your sphere that were not present before. New subtle stresses may have lowered your immune system or your tolerance to certain things. These conditions may be temporary or represent new life conditions you need to work with, and include people, pets and where you spend your time.

Secondly, ask yourself, **Has nothing changed?** If your life appears static, a rare occurrence in my opinion, then perhaps something in your space has crept up on you and is causing a disharmony in your life. It could be your old house is getting moldy and you haven't been down in the basement for a long time to notice. Or it's possible the orchard or farm you live near is spraying with a new herbicide or pesticide? Your street may now carry more traffic resulting in more exhaust or electromagnetic radiation (EMR) pollution. The high tension wires near your home may be carrying more current adding new levels of EMR's to your environment, weakening your immune system in the process. The same may be true of added electronics to your work or home environment like wireless devices. The key here is to think outside the box, look around, examine your life and be more conscious of your environment to see what could be at issue. Innocuous things should not be overlooked, as your unique constitution may be sensitive to something that you are not aware of at this stage in your life.

Purifying on All Levels

This lifetime is a voyage of discovery about ourselves and from Soul's perspective it is a purification process. As a reminder, we are not just purifying our physical bodies, we are purifying on all levels; our emotions, our Causal Body (Karmic Body) and our thoughts, attitudes, and beliefs carried in the Mental Body. So when one area is purified it is a little lighter. Its vibration has increased and so it calls for a similar shift in all of our bodies. As we lighten up on one level, it affects the other parts of us and when we do not make changes, we can eventually fall into a state of disharmony or "dis-ease" in that area. So expect to make changes in order to move forward into a new state of harmony.

Bringing negative energies such as violence into one's life through exposure to certain movies, television programs, music, video games and reading material can have a toxic effect on our subtle bodies – our emotional and mental bodies in particular. The effects of these negative energies act as a pollutant on our being, so be conscious that every person, thing or experience we connect with either purifies or pollutes the body. This includes such influences as foul language, sexual references/behavior, anger/rage, greed or extreme materiality – all of these can exert a downward pull on our well-being, in effect dragging one into a lower consciousness or vibration, setting up disharmonies in the body. Even being exposed to extreme vanity in the form of arrogance or distain can have its effects.

Discovering Apparent Causes

Life can be a puzzle more often than not. What appears to be causing a problem may be a mask for something else. And other issues in life may not appear to have any physical causal origins. This is where you will need to begin to cast your vision in all directions.

Let's start with some basics.

Tobacco and Recreational Drugs: It goes without saying that these substances are obvious toxins and sooner or later will have a negative effect.

Allopathic Medicines: Most prescription or over-the-counter (OTC) drugs are known to have side effects which are really direct effects in your body. By taking a drug you are trading off the greater remediation power of the drug for the perceived lesser effects these can have on your body. So as stated before, be aware that what others can assimilate in their bodies may not be compatible with your body. Drugs typically mask issues. Natural remedies can also mask unless you are actively working with the process to discover what you need to change about yourself.

Your Personal Environment

The areas where you spend your time are critical to your well-being. These include your dwelling, workspace, vehicle and where you spend time with fitness, entertainment, hobbies or sports. Have any of these changed recently? Today's buildings can contain materials for which you could have a sensitivity like paints, carpets, coatings on floors, air quality systems and more. Make a complete assessment of these areas for possible clues to sensitivities you may have. I recently visited a new model home for a housing development. The chemical odours were so bad I had to leave.

At work, do you handle glues, sprays, cleaners, toxins, fertilizers, herbicides, radiation, airport security scanners etc? Many of these modern products are deemed safe, but remember that you are unique. Any product can have an undesirable effect. *Don't judge your body by what others can do.*

The Pest Control Technician

My husband once purchased a fridge from a used appliance shop for a rental unit he owned. It wasn't long before the tenant called telling him there were cockroaches coming out of the fridge. He immediately called a pest control company. When he met the technician he was shocked at how disfigured he was. He had a large boil on his face, one eye was much larger than the other and he walked bent over with a slight limp. He advised my husband to clear the area as he put on a mask and began to spray the nest in the bottom of the fridge. My husband told me, in speaking to him after his spraying, it was clear that he did not associate his conditions with the chemical spray he was using!

The Larger Environment

Your greater environment includes many passive items that could be mildly or totally toxic to your body. These include noise, EMR's (electromagnetic radiation from high tension wires, electronic devices like computers and TVs) and solar radiation. Some feel we are all participating in a giant experiment in involuntary epidemiology — being irradiated by cell phones and towers, cordless phones, satellites, broadcast antennas, military and aviation radar, wireless mice and sound systems, internet, wireless LANs in schools and the workplace, energy saving fluorescent light bulbs and smart meters. And researchers know what it does to some of us. Two experts on these issues are Dr. Dietrich Klinghardt MD, PhD of the Sophia health Institute and the Klinghardt Academy, and Physicist and Microwave Weapons expert, Barrie Trower.

The main problem isn't cancer as it takes a long time to develop. Other problems seem to show up first: neurological, reproductive, and cardiac issues. Also problems with memory loss, severe headaches, sleep disturbances, learning disabilities, attention deficit disorder, and infertility can show up long before cancer. When cancer does appear, it's typically brain tumors, leukemia, and lymphoma. So if you are experiencing any of these issues or symptoms, check your electronics environment. Any one of these influences could be compromising your immune system, or possibly the combination of effects is enough to cause your system to fall into "ill ease." Combine these influences with normal doses of stress and you have a compounded issue. So no one effect may be a cause; it may be a combination that is set off by a trigger like a change in your life that is causing anxiety or stress, or a change in diet.

EMR Precautions

The risks associated with cellular phones and other devices due to electromagnetic radiation (EMR) are emerging globally. Devra Davis, author of *Disconnect* and other experts suggest precautions you can take to avoid health issues including the following:

> Use text features over voice calling and hold the device away from you;
>
> If you must make a voice call, use speaker phone or a wired headset;
>
> If you want to use a wireless headset, do it with a low-power Bluetooth emitter;
>
> Do not carry a phone turned on next to your body;

Use extra care regarding wireless synchronization of hearing aids.

Be cautious of radiation shields that claim to limit exposure to EMR's as they can reduce the connection quality, forcing the phone to transmit at a higher power output. The same applies to signal quality in your location. If low, (e.g. rural area or in an elevator) the weaker signal has to boost itself, increasing your exposure.

When it comes to other serious EMR sources, good alternatives are corded telephones, LED energy saving light bulbs, limiting your exposure to public wireless Internet environments and turning your wireless router off when not in use, which is what I do.

...there is no such thing as a safe dose of radiation, since your risk of genetic and immune-system damage correlates with the total amount of radiation you have received over your lifetime, and any amount, however small, adds to that cumulative total risk. Never believe anyone who tells you that the amount of radiation coming at you from any source is too small to matter.

Andrew Weil, MD, author of 8 Weeks to Optimum Health

Body Products

What you put on your body is almost as important as what you put into your body. Allergens are caused by holding toxins in the body and your skin may be absorbing chemicals from a long list of products that are in common use but which could be the cause of issues for you. Do your own research on the following items and switch to natural or organic if you'd like to test the effects: sunscreen, make-up, body lotion, soap, shampoo, hair colorant, aftershave lotion, hair gels and sprays, perfumes, and deodorant all could contain potentially harmful chemicals to your body.

As a sunscreen or after sun oil, I personally use coconut oil or sesame oil with a blend of essential oils known to protect and nourish the skin. Both coconut and sesame oil have a natural SPF of 15. For body lotion I also use an essential oil blend in almond oil.

Household Products

The following items could also be a source for health issues: fabric softener sheets, air fresheners, stain guard sprays, deodorizer sprays, cleaners, and laundry soaps.

Building Materials

Construction materials and surfaces in your environment are also coming into the limelight as causing problems for some among us. If you have recently renovated or moved into a new home, the following items should not be overlooked. The most common problem sources are: paint, drywall, carpeting, floor finishes, pressure-treated wood, and insulation.

Water Quality

Something to check into? There is a scarcity of clean, fresh water sources on the planet today. Get your water checked for possible toxins, fertilizer, drug residue, bacteria, and unwanted minerals that are present or added.

Fitness and Exercise

Fresh air and exercise are important to good balanced health. How would you rate yourself in this department? Too much or not enough? Both are contributors to an unbalanced physical body.

Clothing

Your clothing can be a source for illness. Don't overlook the effects of modern synthetic fabrics that may stifle your energy or irritate your skin or even transfer an irritant into your body.

Hidden Poisons

There are some harmful poisons in our lives, depending on one's degree of tolerance, that we don't seem to notice and some of these have the potential to cause havoc with our health. The chemicals used in nail care services and products are one such category that could be compromising your health. Another is vaccinations. For example, as Jessica found, many immunizations contain preservatives such as mercury and formaldehyde and surprisingly today, autoimmune diseases are now being traced to vaccinations. Research has also indicated that encephalitis is an acknowledged medical reaction to many vaccinations.

Encephalitis is an acute inflammation of the brain and even a very mild form could lead to personality distortions and disorders. Other symptoms include headache, fever, confusion, drowsiness, and fatigue. More advanced and serious symptoms include seizures or convulsions, tremors, hallucinations, and memory problems.

A review of people surviving the encephalitis epidemics that swept America and Europe in the 1920's revealed that those who survived this condition would suffer from other various issues which were unheard of then but are recognized today as the following: ADD, ADHD, autism, Asperger's syndrome, anorexia, bulimia, impulsive violence, stuttering, mental retardation, dyslexia, sudden infant death syndrome, processing disorders, allergies, bed-wetting, Tourette's seizures, and sexual identity disorders.

Mercury, a Big Problem

Reflecting back on Jessica's experience, we can see mercury is a particular concern. It has a very strong ability to mess up your entire system, which is part of the reason why mercury toxicity symptoms are so difficult to pin down. For example, some symptoms even relate to anxiety and depression. Mercury seems to have four main sources: dental amalgam fillings, vaccines, fish consumption and mercury pollution from coal-burning power plants. Ask yourself what your exposure is or has been to these four areas.

If you are experiencing any of the diseases or conditions mentioned above, you may wish to look into having a heavy metals test. If positive, check out the benefits of detoxification cleanses and chelation therapy (intravenous is the most effective). There are several methods that a doctor, naturopath or homeopath can assist with. There may also be lifestyle and dietary changes that can assist to reduce your exposure to harmful chemicals and metals to your body type.

Heavy Metal Toxicity: Common Symptoms
You may have heavy metal toxicity if you are experiencing any of these symptoms:

- Chronic pain throughout the muscles and tendons or any soft tissues of the body;
- Chronic malaise – general feeling of discomfort, fatigue, and illness;
- Brain fog – state of forgetfulness and confusion;
- Chronic infections such as Candida;
- Gastrointestinal complaints, such as diarrhea, constipation, bloating, gas, heartburn, and indigestion;
- Food allergies;
- Dizziness;
- Migraines and/or headaches;
- Visual disturbances;
- Mood swings, depression, and/or anxiety;
- Nervous system malfunctions – burning extremities, numbness, tingling, paralysis, and/or an electrifying feeling throughout the body.

Material World Check-list

The key to discovering causes of imbalance and irritation in your material world is to open up to all the possibilities, to audit every corner of your life for possible areas that may be causing or contributing to issues. Keep in mind that this journey may call for change of some kind, not only in the physical environment, but in other areas of your life... to be explored in the coming chapters.

Review Your Life

Review this list of items and rate yourself on how these could be affecting your health:

Fitness: Are you getting enough exercise to keep you healthy and to de-stress?

Water: Are you drinking enough? Do you know what your water contains? Do you have a purification system?

Work: Exposure to obvious toxins and chemicals?

Air quality: Workplace location such as a sealed office tower.

Building materials: Carpeting, drywall, insulation, pressure-treated lumber and paints can be the source of issues.

Vehicle: Do you sit in traffic? Do you make long commutes?

Home: Have you inspected your residence recently?

Are there new building materials present?

Has there been any asbestos removed such as old floor tile?

How old is your furnace? Has it been checked for gas leaks?

Is your residence near or downwind from a busy road, farm, high tension wires, or factory (pollution, EMR)?

Soils: Some can contain lead and radon gas? This may be a problem source for gardeners and children.

EMR Electromagnetic radiation is causing issues among some people. How do you use your mobile device? Text or voice calling? Where do you carry your phone? Do you protect yourself from EMR while at your computer? Do you live or work near EMR sources like transformers, transmission wires, wireless devices and radio broadcast antennas?

Do you use cordless home phones?

Sun Tanning: Do you use a tanning salon? Is their equipment the latest technology?

Clothing: How do you feel in your present clothing choices? I suggest that you monitor this area as it is a subtle area that could be the source or contributor to a compound issue.

Body Products: Make a review of these.

Household Products and Cleaners: Review these as well.

Exposure to heavy metals such as mercury and lead.

My Life Environment Today
Here's a snapshot of my life at present.

Entertainment influences: Mostly reality and how-to television with National Geographic and OWN (Oprah), with some HGTV added. My reading material is spiritual, health, fitness, yoga, Pilates, aromatherapy, and reflexology and inspirational. The movies I see are usually romantic comedy or light action adventure.

Spiritual practices: I have a daily half hour contemplation with my husband every evening after dinner. My reading material will often be a personal growth book on spiritual principles. The combination of contemplation, spiritual reading and being open to the nudges and inspiration of spirit is also key for me. Giving service to others is also vital to my spiritual growth.

Giving back: I love helping others through fitness, massage, reflexology and in understanding key spiritual concepts.

Exercise: I teach Pilates, yoga, strength and cardio training and personal train others 10 to 12 hours a week, walk our dog and also play pickleball, golf and ski. I find that it's important for me to work out on my own at home incorporating burst training into my routine three times per week.

General lifestyle: I like to wear natural materials. We cook with stainless steel, store left-over's in glass, and use the microwave only for heating up heating pads. In the summer, I preserve fresh picked fruits and vegetables which we enjoy all year.

Communications: I have shifted to using my cell phone on speaker held away from my body. I try to use a land line wherever possible while at home or working. I do not use cordless phones and we use our Wi-Fi sparingly for our tablet (it has an on-off switch).

Making Conscious Choices: My Top Suggestions

Current Choice	Issue	Conscious Choice
Cordless Phone	Electromagnetic Radiation (EMR)	Land Line
Cell phone	EMR	Texting, Speaker Phone
Fluorescent light bulbs	EMR	LED Light Bulbs
Wireless Networks	EMR	Wired Connections
Hi-tension Wires	EMR	Avoid
Microwave Towers	EMR	Avoid
Medicines	Toxicity	Natural, Nutritious Foods
Glues/Sprays/Cleaners	Toxicity	Natural Products
Fertilizers	Toxicity	Natural/Compost
Body/Make-up	Toxicity	Natural Products
Deodorant	Toxicity	Natural Products
Perfume	Toxicity	Aromatherapy Oils
Nail Care Products	Toxicity	Natural Products
Immunizations	Mercury	Nutritious Foods
Tuna, Fish	Mercury	Fresh Fish
Water	Metals & Drug Residue	R.O. Purification

The doctor of the future will give no medicine but will interest his patients in the care of the human frame, in diet, and in the cause and prevention of disease.

Thomas Edison

Now let's take a look at the effect our emotions can have on our health.

4

Outgrow Emotional Toxins

I find that resentment, criticism, guilt and fear cause more problems than anything else. These four things cause the major problems in our bodies and in our lives. These feelings come from blaming others and not taking responsibility for our own experiences.

Louise Hay, You Can Heal Your Life

Therese's Story

Therese is a fellow yoga teacher and Reiki practitioner and viewed herself as a calm, balanced and peaceful individual. However, one day a few years ago she found herself in excruciating pain with a sciatic nerve problem. As a yoga teacher this was a major challenge. She told me, "I was in pain all the time," she told me and had difficulty moving. She finally found she had to stop teaching. For two years she lived with the pain but she was on a search for the reason. She was doing everything she could do to deal with it. She told me, "the pain was running down my leg and I could hardly walk. I was trying yoga to stretch it out, I was icing it, I was seeing a chiropractor, even taking aspirin to sleep at night, and I was trying to figure it out from a spiritual standpoint in my meditations. I was asking myself what was out-of-balance in my life. It was at this two-year point that I surrendered to God, and in that act of surrender I could feel the energy coming in. I went into a healing cycle after that.

"I began to follow a cookie crumb trail and it led me to a book written by a medical doctor. The book said I had to talk to my sciatic nerve. The author said that in his experience with thousands of patients that eighty per cent of back pain is psychosomatic and involved emotions. Shortly thereafter I found myself at a friend's dinner party and ended up talking to a spiritual fellow from India. After about ten minutes of chit chat, he said to me: 'You have a lot of anger in you.' I was floored. I turned to my good friend and asked her, 'do I have anger in me?' She said, 'of course not. You are a wonderful person.' Nevertheless, he said he felt a lot of anger. I denied this judgement at first, but his comment stuck with me.

"After that experience, a yoga teacher friend suggested I see a man who did emotional release work. In our session, he asked a lot of questions, particularly about people in my life. He combined his questions with kinesiology (muscle testing) and it was showing I was testing weak for several people – the men in my life! That realization sent me down the road of forgiveness – forgiving the men and then forgiving myself for not standing in my truth.

"Within two days of that session, all the pain disappeared! I suddenly could walk normally. The pain has never come back. If I feel a twinge, I talk to my back saying; 'I'm not going to allow you to seize up on me again. I am going to deal with my emotions and not let them have an impact on my body.'

Shortly after the healing, Therese was motivated to take a weekend course in New York on being more aware of her emotions. She confided, "this course revealed for me that I had blocked emotions in my body; I had to learn about when I was blocking and stifling, and when an emotion was a negative one. In this pivotal weekend I learned to identify emotions and figure out a way to release them in a healthy way, giving love to myself and to my world.

Developing a Stronger Connection with Spirit

"Throughout this discovery process I felt my connection to Spirit was guiding me through a process of healing during my meditations, helping me move forward with my life, revealing to me what I needed to do to move forward pain-free. The process gave me a feeling of incredible love and I could also feel a lot of energy. When I truly surrendered that day, that's when everything speeded up. My healing came in three weeks and for me I had experienced a miracle.

"One of my most significant moments was when that Indian stranger said, 'You are an angry person.' It was such an out-of-the-blue comment; it pushed me to go in a new direction. When he said it, it was highlighted. I felt that his words were illuminated with lights – that there was a message for me.

Taking it to a Higher Level

Therese was initially doing everything she could think of to help herself such as yoga, chiropractic treatments and massage, but she needed to change the focus of her search to a higher level of exploration. "I attribute a lot of my success solving this health puzzle from doing Reiki II, a type of healing on myself, and in the process I was writing down feelings and impressions which were helping me connect," she told me. "When I did the absent healings, it connected me with my higher self for guidance. I was examining who I was."

"Most importantly, I had to have humility to change my self-beliefs. I thought of myself as this wonderful, kind, peaceful person but underneath all of this was anger. I needed help to see it. I had to look at myself as human and admit I had this anger; I wasn't this divine serene being I imagined I was. I had to see I had some negative traits – I was not as loving and peaceful as I had thought. So I needed humility to get down on my knees to ask God for help.

"There was a huge shift in me!

Spiritual Realizations Flood In

"I've discovered a new level of compassion for others going through a human experience in this healing process. It's given me so much understanding for others and a huge love and respect for it. I feel such gratitude for this life where I can grow, learn and expand."

When I asked Therese if she has discovered a new spiritual awareness operating in her life, she replied, "I now recognize that I have come here to be joy. I can see my purpose a lot clearer now. When I get out of harmony, out of balance, I lose consciousness of who I am and I am no longer fulfilling my purpose of being joy.

"I have also needed to learn detachment – detachment from the belief and image I had constructed of myself. I believed I was this peaceful being which was not true. I had to let go of this false image that I had created and believed to be true, accept who I truly am and to love myself. You see, my whole life was image (Therese was an actor earlier in life). It wasn't real. I had to be authentic, honest and learn. I had to ask myself, 'what am I truly feeling?'"

∞

What is Emotion?

More often than not, our emotions are so much a part of us that we cannot see them in their true light. A part of our journey into good health and personal growth in this lifetime is recognizing patterns of behaviour that are integral to our being and their consequent emotional components. Emotions that are no longer serving us are at the center of many disharmonies in our bodies and can be the cause of disease in their extreme manifestation.

Emotion is energy in motion (e-motion). It excites, stirs, and agitates our feelings and, like Therese discovered, can either contribute to our upliftment or the degradation of our harmony. Our emotions can be beneficial like laughter, or counterproductive to our being like anger. Should we harbour an emotion for a period of time that runs counter to our overall constitution, an aberration can develop. Then there is a part of us that is not in harmony with the whole. The severity of the gap between our overall harmony or vibration and the feeling of disharmony, will determine our overall state of balance or imbalance.

Theses disharmonies have then found a place of residence in our bodies and can become visible as discomfort, illness, a condition or an abnormality. Some of the most common negative emotions that can affect us are fear, hate, sorrow or grief, and worry.

Fear Shuts Out Love

The emotion of fear and the emotional anxiety it brings shuts out love, trust and creativity. It is a most destructive emotion that can stop us in our tracks from moving forward. Our destiny (as Soul having a human lifetime) may want to take us into new situations, relationships, careers - activities for its growth and learning, but fear has the power to halt this progress. The result can be manifested as an internal conflict reflected in the body. This can make itself known as a minor condition at first but then become a full blown challenge.

Most "dis-ease" (disharmony) follows a pattern of progression. First the imbalance is known at higher levels, perhaps felt in the heart as a knowingness. But as this heart-feeling is ignored and the imbalance or desire to follow Soul's agenda is suppressed by a fear, the situation may then present itself as a conscious awareness or thought. Ignoring these thoughts then can translate into the physical body. Further suppression of the issue via medical or natural interventions may forestall the condition but there may be an eventual level of seriousness that manifests, Soul's way of getting us to listen to its message.

Many conditions can be brought under control by being aware of this process of manifestation of disharmonies. If something does not feel right, the disharmony can be corrected by making changes. So the body "talks" to us, and our emotions therefore are a key to good health.

One such outcome of fear is a lack of flexibility. This can reflect in the body as a stiff neck as I have discovered on my own life-adventure. Today, whenever I feel stiffness in a joint or in my neck, I ask myself where my inflexibility is coming from. Or, how gracefully am I accepting a change?

"Whatever happens in our emotional body also occurs in our physical body...Through the mind-body connection, any repressed feelings of wanting and deserving harmony, peace, stability, and a simple sense of joy in life are translated into appropriate bio-chemical responses in the body. This effectively deprives the body cells of all these positive qualities as well."

"Whatever you keep to yourself out of fear of being criticized or hurt, actually turns into poisons in the body."

Andreas Moritz, *Cancer is Not a Disease, It's a Survival Mechanism*

Love, the Antidote to Fear

The antidote to fear is love. Fear cannot exist where there is love. Embodied in love is confidence and trust. Our lesson plan, our life path may be calling for us to grow beyond the false limitations of fear. Our anxieties may be hidden in such things as resisting changes; we may feel we are comfortable where we are, but are we really resisting out of deeply embedded trepidation? We are being stretched beyond our comfort zone. An honest examination of one's self is required here, exploring the hidden aspects of our nature, something we may not want to open up. This may reveal a hidden fear of failure, or of loss, for example.

Often, we are ready for something new such as a new setting, or for a change in relationships, career, residence and more. Love in a spiritual sense is all about trusting that there is good in all change. The expression, "It's all good" sums this up succinctly.

But how does one conquer fear. First by recognizing that it is fear that is inhibiting your movement forward into the future. Second, by asking for help in conquering the fear and accepting the change. Third, by taking action.

Yvonne's Story

When Yvonne was young she was told her knees would deteriorate and give her problems later in life. And so a couple of years ago when her knee stiffened and then became painful, she knew she would have to face this challenge and do something about it. It was bone on bone rubbing, and very painful. Yvonne recalled, "For two years I put it off. I felt I could fix it. During this time, I could feel the fears emerging inside me. I was thinking, what if things went wrong? What would happen if the surgery failed and I couldn't walk afterward? How could a failed operation be corrected?" Yvonne was gripped in this fearful consciousness and couldn't get above these emotions. "The negative was stronger than the positive at this time, yet I knew deep down that it would be very negative for me if I let this fear grip me for a long time.

"I finally went to see my doctor and then a specialist who told me I needed knee replacement surgery. It turned out I knew the specialist surgeon. We had connected many years before, so he was not a complete stranger to me. This was a comfort to me and calmed my fears down somewhat. I understood I had to have the surgery in spite of my doubts and worries. I knew then I could do this."

Listening, a Key to Acceptance

Yvonne continued, "In the process of acceptance of the reality of surgery, I had to learn to listen only to the positive and I had to learn to be quiet: I also realized how powerful quietness is. When I had questions, I'd tune inward or simply read a book title and then sit quietly, and I could feel my fear subside in the silence with no outside world buzz. Contemplation helped me open inner doors. This became my journey.

"A turning point for me in accepting the operation and moving beyond my fears was a dream I experienced. In the dream, my inner guidance told me I was going to be OK. I was sensing quietness and love at the same time, and it was a beautiful feeling.

"After my acceptance and surrender, everything I needed was coming to me in a natural way. I was open to messages. As a result, the rest was like a journey that was all arranged for me. One day I received an inspiration in my daily contemplation that I needed to work on my whole body before the operation; I needed to get much stronger and get in shape. When I came to that conclusion I was serendipitously connected with a personal trainer through a friend. I knew this is because I had surrendered to Spirit. The trainer had extensive experience working with people who were recovering from knee and hip replacement operations. And so I was able to exercise my core and knee before the operation, for knee surgery was major – it was a new body part like getting a new heart part. So part of accepting the surgery was accepting my new body part. I knew I'd have to like my new knee.

"I remember going into surgery and had no memories after that and woke up with my new knee. I looked down at the bandage and said, 'I have a new friend.' I was accepting it. At times I cried after the operation for no reason. On one occasion I asked, 'What have I done?' As I sobbed, a nurse heard me and spoke some words of understanding, validating my emotions over letting it all go. That helped me move on and I never cried again. I transitioned to accepting my new knee like a friend. I was walking again without pain." Yvonne likened the feeling by saying, "It's like getting a new heart. It's not yours. There is an acceptance needed."

Writing it All Down

Yvonne's journaling played a major role in her speedy recovery. "Writing in my journal, I could feel the love of the gift of a new knee. I discovered through my writing I had to learn how to receive, how to accept something that isn't mine. I questioned myself: 'Why did I get it? Why am I supposed to have it?' And the answer came: 'It's what I need now.' I realized I tend to fight the idea of being deserving - accepting. I'm a caregiver – I would help others. This time the role was reversed. I had to be accepting, not giving. I had to learn how to receive love, and in the process, how to love myself. I realized I needed this in order to give love."

Before the operation, one of my fears was stairs. I expressed this to the doctor and he assured me he would ensure post operative training for stairs. But I still went ahead and arranged all of my furniture on the main level of my home so I could have one-floor living and not have to use the stairs. When I got home after the operation, I looked at the stairs and went straight up! I actually was doing stairs better than walking. It was a mind thing. I had to move past the mind.

Today I'm more aware of what I eat. I'm aware of my weight and I'm more in tune with the vegan way of eating. I'm trying not to abuse my knee. It's making me more conscious of taking care of myself so I can take care of my knee.

Key Lessons on the Way

Yvonne learned many valuable lessons on her journey. "I learned how fear can creep into your life, like the fear of having to depend on others, but knowledge helped me overcome it. I'm more trusting now; the process taught me to trust and become quiet. Life is very, very peaceful for me.

"My nature is to find humor in things, but I lost it for a while when I was in fear. Having a strong spiritual focus in my life made life a little easier. It gave me a live-in-the-moment attitude, to just let it be.

"I've learned more about detachment – not to be so attached because these things can be taken away. I lost my knee, but got a new one. I say, accept what you get given back to you. It may not be the same thing – be thankful.

"I'm grateful for these medical gifts we have today. I now look at people and surroundings the same way, with gratefulness. My knee got me through another go around – I couldn't walk – I was given another so I can move on with my life."

Yvonne knows now. "These things are written in your destiny," she counsels. "There is a reason. So accept. Live through it, then you are on the other side of it – and changed in the process. I find it's now easier to accept the bumps in the road and keep going. I say thank you for the experience. Learn to love. Roll with the punch – you can get through anything. Don't abuse what you are given."

Yvonne's final word: "Love what you are given. Love the gifts in life. I'll have two as I'm having my other knee done as well. Learn to accept and love whatever you are given. Everything is positive in life. My knee has healed so fast, it's like I never had a problem!"

∞

Conquering Fear with Contemplation

In dealing with fear, the most powerful tool I can suggest is contemplation. It helps me make that important inner connection and get above the problems of the day.

I sit comfortably in an easy chair, close my eyes and gently place my attention on the screen of my imagination, a point just above and between my eyebrows. Then I think of something I love. I've found fear cannot exist where love is present. (I'll delve more into contemplation in a later chapter.)

∞

Most of us are around people constantly who have tension, fear, headaches, deafness, rheumatism, illnesses, reserve and unwillingness to accept others as friends, heart troubles, timidity and reluctance to face the world. ...The problem here is simply tension.

What causes tension? It is really fear.

Paul Twitchell, The Flute of God

Sorrow and Disharmony

The second of the emotional downfalls is sorrow or grief. Grief causes a serious negative disharmony in our being if left too long. We need to allow ourselves a reasonable amount of time to heal from any loss whether it is the loss of a loved one, the loss of a job or even the loss of our financial security. Healing from these losses can follow the five stages of grief and healing from loss that Elizabeth Kubler-Ross defined: denial, anger, bargaining, depression, and acceptance. The first four components of this process are a negative drain on our harmony and can occur in any order, can be revisited or be wrapped up in a package of grief. This grief, left unattended can sap your energy, shut down your heart keeping you from love, and this can manifest as disease. Sadness and feeling down are other negative aspects of this emotional state.

My husband told me that one of his greatest challenges in recent years was serving as a hospice volunteer, helping patients and their loved ones deal with anticipated loss and actual loss. One key learning he took away from his three years in this volunteer service was to empower patients and those close to them. In this process there seemed to be inherent in the experience a willingness to address feelings, to get them out into full expression. He told me he could see that this was more helpful in moving through the loss than not acknowledging the feelings, hanging on to them, prolonging the grieving process.

Moving into Healing from Grief

With the help of others, you can learn from your experience and move forward. In this process you gain greater strength to conquer all challenges. Through the process of loss one is learning empathy, surrender, acceptance, gratitude and many other qualities. As in tackling fear, contemplation can be a wonderful tool to use to connect you with your highest perspective, helping you heal from your loss in a genuine way.

Worry and Stress

If you are focussed on the past, you can tend to be regretful or remorseful. If your attention is on the future, you can feel worry which will result in stress. By this I mean that if your thoughts are dominated by what *may* happen, then you are creating a condition of worry and causing stress in your body. This emotion can be very damaging to your health over time. The key here is to recognize where you are. Do you lament the past, what could have been, what you could have done better? Are you thinking about what could happen or that something might not go well? The key is to find middle ground, the present moment.

If you are putting your attention in the past or future, perhaps you can find the present. It can be a very calm place. The future has not occurred, and the past can be forgotten, water over the dam so to speak. Try to find that present moment of contentment. Contemplation can help you to place your attention in the present moment and to fill your "present" with love.

To be in the present, you have to be in a position to enjoy every moment. If your life is a series of destinations connected by travel time in between, chances are you are rushing through life and giving yourself a great deal of disease-causing tension in the process. The key is to slow down and live the transition time as in-the-moment time. Slow your driving, slow your walking down, and leave more time to get places so you can relax - even plan on arriving early!

The Five Channels of Self-Destruction and Illness

We are on our own life-path and this is occurring on several levels – physical, emotional, karmic, mental and spiritual; often, health and healing is a journey into higher levels of awareness that is linked to changes in consciousness. Our harmonious make-up is a moving target as we grow in awareness, conscious realizations and elevate our vision of who we are providing us with some key personal lessons.

These lessons center around five channels or behaviours that have a negative pole and a positive pole. The negative pole represents the lowest attributes of the human condition, and the opposite pole is our goal, spiritual perfection and clarity of the human condition. At the positive pole, we have reached a point of total service to all life; we are dedicated to helping others in their life journey.

These five channels of growth exist for everyone and, in this present moment, we each have our own place within these channels somewhere between the poles.

The five negative poles are defined as lust (self-indulgence), anger, greed, vanity and attachment.

The five positive poles are: discrimination (making right choices), forgiveness, contentment, humility and detachment.

Companion Emotions of the Five Channels

These five channels carry with them companion emotions that can be the source of illness and an opportunity for improved health. They represent a continuum for our growth and we find ourselves living in these channels as we go about our daily living. How we interact with others is the key, and by understanding these channels, we can see where our current position is and what may be underlying a state of dis-ease or illness. Our personal health is tied directly to these five channels in the human condition. Because we are on this life-path of personal growth, these channels within us need to be purified and if one channel is out of step or balance with our total being or consciousness, it can cause illness.

These channels have an influence on all of the bodies we carry: the physical, emotional, causal and mental. At this moment, let's take a look at the emotional body influences these channels hold.

1. Lust (Self-indulgence): Indulging One's Own Desires Without Restraint

Lust is having an abnormal appetite for drugs, alcohol, tobacco, highly spiced foods, fatty foods, sweets, highly processed snack foods and sex. Some manifestations in human behaviour are gluttony, reading obscene material, and self-gratification.

Other manifestations are an abnormal appetite for money, power, things, and recognition, and these imbalances may sow the seeds of disharmony in our body. This can show up in a person as being self-centered and uncaring of others. It places one at the low end of the scale of human evolution - **the opposite pole being discrimination and balance** - making right choices. Somewhere between these two poles you will find yourself.

Sooner or later, your life journey will take you another step closer to the positive polarity and these behaviours, however mild will need purification. Taking another step forward will be necessary.

2. Anger: My Way or the Highway

Anger stirs up trouble and represents an extreme position of, "I want it my way." Anger says, "This is not what I want," and, "I'm not flexible." It is resistance to the way things have unfolded. So as such, anger is an extreme form of resistance to the flow of life and could be a major source of imbalance.

Anger creates hatred and causes emotional burn-out. Jealously, malice and resentment are companion negative emotions that are fuelled by anger, one's resistance to the way life is unfolding at that time. Milder forms of anger include annoyance, brooding, irritation, being ticked-off, agitation and impatience.

Being dismissive with another person, their ideas or their behaviours, or, anger at a situation that may feel like a loss of face, has a habit of affecting the angry one profoundly. Other behavioural aspects of anger include slander, gossip, profanity, faultfinding, peevishness, mockery and ill will.

Anger is an impediment to harmony and clouds the mind, and it is usually expressed in a harsh way which destroys relationships. (Anger can also be expressed as a simmering silence.)

All anger, even in its milder forms has the potential to manifest as illness, and uncontrolled anger over a period of time can manifest as deep-seated disease. (Reflect back on Therese's issue with her sciatic nerve.) Some say that depression is anger turned inward. Others link cancer to anger and describe cancer like a war going on in the body, a struggle between what the mind wants and what the heart is seeking. As indicated above, anger can take some very mild forms so you need to be aware of these aspects that may need to change at your place in life.

The polar opposite of anger in this channel is forgiveness and tolerance. This is a key area for examination in your life. When something occurs in your life that has the potential to cause you anger or one of the milder forms of it such as irritation, frustration or annoyance, the faster you can rebalance into forgiveness or tolerance, the better off you are.

3.   Greed and its Many Forms

Greed fixes us to the materialistic things of life such as money and its surrogates. It is an extreme focus on attaining and maintaining wealth. It shows its ugly face as miserliness, being stingy, a lack of sharing, deception and trickery.

Subtle forms of greed can manifest as fibs, distortions and "little white lies" which usually have the goal of getting something at the expense of another. It often can involve emotional manipulation and emotional blackmail.

The positive polarity is being content with one's life and financial condition. Know that we have earned our condition in life through our past behaviors, and that in life we need to see that everything we have must be earned either through work, service or by being paid for. There is no fast track through greed to wealth, as this self-destructive behavior will eventually result in an unbalancing in the physical body or at some other level in our being.

The Polar Opposite of Greed is Contentment.

Are you content with your life, within your own skin?

Are you happy to share what you have?

Do you give freely of yourself?

It is difficult to see the many manifestations of greed that could be a part of our character, being immersed in this Western society. The best way to take an objective viewpoint is to look at your ability to give freely, serving others. How sharing are you?

Do you give freely with no strings attached, or do you attach an expectation of reciprocity to your giving, or an expectation of love or friendship?

4. Vanity Has its Disguises

Vanity at the emotional level manifests as egotism, the overgrown opinion of one's self. Behavioural manifestations are arrogance, haughtiness or pride. Vain people can be quite sensitive to criticism. Being a control freak is another hallmark of vanity or pride.

This negative channel that we find ourselves within can also manifest with us in an excessive focus on our physical appearance, pride or a preoccupation with how we think others see us. Some manifestations could be over attention given to position, title, cars we drive, clothing we wear and our neighbourhood, or size of house. Some of the behaviours that flow from vanity are bragging, faultfinding and scolding, pride and haughtiness. Vanity in its extreme form has an expression in the need to punish those who oppose us.

Remember that you are a unique being and at this stage in your spiritual growth, these aspects of vanity may be very subtle. The key words here are "over attention."

Vanity can also take the form of "spiritual vanity", in this case letting the emotions or thoughts and beliefs rule over the heart, the gateway to Soul. When the emotions and thoughts rule, we close off our heartfelt desires, our true inner nature. Spiritual vanity ignores the whisperings of the higher Self in favour of reactions that feed the ego, the material being. By this I mean that you may not be following your spiritual nudges, intuitions or other forms of guidance, or you are not maintaining your spiritual connection by giving yourself enough space in your day. In other words you may be underutilizing your spiritual connection by getting caught up in your emotions or your thoughts, and this is also a form of vanity.

This arrogance can be destructive to one's overall harmony and manifest as being ill-at-ease in some way.

Humility is the polar opposite quality we strive for as conscious beings on the road of life. Examples of humility include:

Modesty, a desire to not seek credit;

A willingness to listen to others without a need to share our views;

Not having to be right or convince others of our position or our truth;

Wanting to serve or help others on their terms and to be yielding.

5.   Attachment Offers One More Opportunity for Growth

As with all things in life, there is always one more step on the path of life. This channel of self destruction and poor health involves the *unnecessary* attachment to anything in this materialistic world, as well as to emotions, thought patterns and beliefs.

Attachment fixes us to the lower values of life including our surroundings, associations and relationships with others. It involves placing false values on the trappings of life such as home, position, possessions, vehicle one drives etc. and leads to emotional conditions like worry and anxiety. They say the top worry of wealthy people is the loss of money. Fear of loss rears its head again!

Attachment can also be present in rigidity of thoughts and beliefs, representing inflexibilities which can inhibit our spiritual growth.

Contentment with our life, our families, our things – what we own - is the polar opposite of attachment. This is a consciousness of knowing that everything we have is for our personal growth. The things of life are but props that are to be moved on and off our stage of life to allow us to move through different scenes that are set for our learning. Holding on to our current stage setting can have the effect of stifling our growth.

How easily do you let go of the things in your life, emotions and thought patterns that may no longer be serving your best interests?

Ask Yourself....

Are you hanging on to relationships, social positions, or a job?

Do you consider that the things you have are on loan from Spirit?

Do you understand that to receive something new into your life, you have to make room for it by letting go of other things that are no longer needed?

How easily can you let go of unnecessary things and move on?

What is the degree of clutter in your home, office or life in general? There is a relationship between all these areas, and clutter in one area can affect the free flowing energy in another area of your life.

The opposite pole on the Attachment scale is Detachment, a state of being non-attached to things, people, honours, position, residence and more. It is a state of allowing these physical attributes to flow through our lives as stage decorations or props for our life's lesson plan and the people we are meant to interact with and learn from in a spiritual sense. The easier we can flow through situations and their physical elements, the more we can grow and maintain excellent health.

Detachment also implies flexibility, being open to new ideas and having a willingness to make changes outside our comfort zone.

Making Emotional Changes

This chapter on searching the emotional body has only provided some ideas on the effects of emotions on your physical body. It will involve a process over time of peeling back the layers. To get you started with an honest examination of where you can move forward in your emotional make-up, try the following self-evaluation exercise.

Making Conscious Emotional Choices:

On each line, note where you can take a new step into greater harmony along your path to optimum health.

Negative Pole	A Step I Can Take	Conscious Choice
Fear		**Love**
Fears in my life		Love in my Life

Holding back, Timid	Adventurous
Doubts, Reticence	Confidence
Grief and Sorrow	**Happiness and Joy**
Sadness, Feeling Down, Depression	Enthusiasm for Life
Dealing with grief	Feeling Love of Spirit
Lust	**Discrimination**
Seeking Power and Authority	Serving Others
Self-centered	Caring
Anger	**Forgiveness**
Irritation, Dismissive	Respect
Impatience	Tolerance
Greed	**Contentment**
Stingy, Miserly	Giving Without Conditions
Deceptions, Fibs, Little White Lies	Truth, Open, Honest
Emotional Manipulation	Purity, Kindness
Vanity	**Humility**
Ego, Arrogance	Empowering Others
Control Freak	Relaxed, Creative
Spiritual Vanity	Following Your Heart
Attachment	**Detachment**
Worry, Anxiety	Letting go, finding center
Jealously, Envy	Acceptance
Defined by People,	Defined by interests, values
Position, Possessions	Service to others

There are 3 key emotions that help us heal ourselves:

1) Forgiveness – emotional forgiveness liberates us from the past, especially all the worrying of the past (i.e resentment);

2) Gratitude – when we live in gratitude every day, we're constantly thankful for what we have. Gratitude allows us to move away from the future and gets us back into the present by appreciating what we have;

3) Love – The most powerful emotion that we have is the emotion of love. The emotion of love allows us to really accept ourselves for who we truly are. Love yourself first.

Dr. Fabrizio Mancini

From an interview on his book, The Power of Self-Healing

Now let's take our journey of making more conscious choices into the mind-body arena of thought patterns and beliefs.

5

What You Believe,
You Can Achieve

Attitudes and beliefs...influence how well your food is digested and how effective your exercise is. You have, within you, the power to create a life of joy, abundance, and health, or you have the same ability to create a life filled with stress, fatigue, and disease. With very few exceptions, the choice is yours.

Cristiane Northrup, MD, The Wisdom of Menopause

Ryan's Story

Sandi has been a class student of mine for a number of years. When I heard what happened to her son Ryan, I just knew his experience would be a perfect illustration of this chapter's theme, what you believe, you can achieve.

Two years ago at age fourteen Ryan had landed in Children's Hospital fighting for his life with third degree burns to his face, neck, shoulders, hands and arms. The day started out as one filled with adventure with his buddies, on a hike to a canyon with an amazing waterfall. They had hiked up to the canyon and then used a rope to ascend a two-hundred-and-fifty foot drop to the canyon floor, quite an adventure for fourteen-year-olds.

Ryan described himself and his friends as "a bunch of pyromaniacs." They built a small fire at the bottom to celebrate. They had the fire lit, barely, and they wanted to juice up the flames. As Ryan held a dimly lit torch, his friend held a water bottle full of gasoline. Ryan asked his friend to spray some gas on the torch. Their adventure suddenly turned to horror!

Ryan was engulfed in a whoosh of gas-fired flames and the brush behind him even caught fire. Here is what happened in his own words: "I took off running and for twenty seconds I was trying to pat out the flames and get them off my face, neck and chest. Running only accelerated the flames. My friend told me to get in the river, but I hesitated because I knew it was glacial. However, I was in so much severe pain, I jumped in. The frigid water cooled the flames out. When I came back to my friends they saw half my face was missing! My face, hands and neck were severely burned – it looked like my body was skinned. My lungs and throat were also singed. With so much adrenalin going, I wrapped my hands in cloth and, using the rope, scaled up the two-hundred-fifty-foot canyon wall to the top. My friend called his sister who came and drove us to the hospital."

In the hospital Ryan's singed throat began to swell shut and he entered into critical condition. He was stabilized and air ambulanced to a major Children's Hospital. During the next three days, Ryan faced life and death issues including low blood pressure and then a bad lung infection. At this point, he began to lose his fight to live. "I felt tired, defeated and was living with mild sedation and a breathing tube stuck down my neck," he recounted. "My situation was weighing on me."

Awakening to a Higher Consciousness of Being

"A few days later when the tube came out I had a profound experience – an awakening of gratitude. Even though my face looked like a pig's ear dog treat, I reached an acceptance of my condition and that I was not going to die. I felt an amazing appreciation for listening to music, drinking water again, having a chocolate shake – everything became so peaceful for me. It was awesome to breathe without that tube. I felt deep gratitude for all the little things and for being alive – I was excited to be alive versus just being in a body!"

Now it was time for Ryan to heal. Ryan spent six days in the hospital and then was sent home to live in a sterile environment. He had weekly journeys back to the hospital for the next four weeks. Ryan was told he would need skin grafts to repair the severe damage, yet as I saw Ryan eighteen months later, he had no visible signs of the burns!

A Positive Attitude

Ryan explained, "I never let the idea of getting an infection or having any other issues even enter my mind. I deeply believed this could not happen and that I would heal normally. I held a very positive outlook. I had a saying, 'I'm going to have such a healing day. These scars are going to just fade away.' I didn't see myself as being too physically changed. I thought myself well. In spite of what I was told, I never bought into how bad it could be. I would put on music and meditate/contemplate and see myself well. I would intend – watching my skin repair – kinda like mindfulness. I maintained this level of inspiration and hope."

It was during the healing months that Ryan was introduced to a spiritual woman by a family friend. He told me, "I just knew we had met in a past life. When I went into her shop, I was so drawn to her.

She looked at me and told me I have a healing vibe. We became friends very quickly and I trusted her. Since our meeting, all of my wisdom has come from her – she answers a lot of my questions. She's been a catalyst for my spiritual evolution and I speak to her every few days. She's like a mentor.

A New Passion for Serving Others

"Shortly after meeting her, I was attracted to Reiki (a form of therapy where the practitioner channels energy into a patient to encourage healing) after being introduced to it by a buddy. Reiki felt like meeting an old friend. It has come naturally and I felt like I had done this a lot in past lives."

Ryan told me, "We exist physically and Reiki is like energetic water – it works on all four levels: physically, emotionally, mentally and spiritually. Reiki is humble. It is not associated with any religion. Whenever I have a 'dis-ease' on any of the four levels, I'll give myself a session. So my healing process from the burns has led me to Reiki and my understanding of reality now – the nature of reality. I connect with this. I'm even building a Reiki room in our house.

"I'm on a journey of uncovering. I now see the light and love in everyone. I see things as they are, and people as they are. I'm no better than anyone else."

Ryan's awakening has affected his whole family who have now discovered contemplation/meditation and are supporting Ryan with his spiritual choices and explorations.

Ryan says his daily meditations/contemplations have helped him immensely. "When I contemplate, I have this knowingness. I just feel it to validate it. I'm trying to go with the experiential aspect to get at truth. I like a lot of the words Buddha spoke about experiencing it for yourself as opposed to religious doctrine. I do a lot of visualization and with healing on the four levels, I use it experientially. We have this persona, but I release this and just experience a true nature of reality."

When I asked Ryan if he had received guidance, intuition, insights or a feeling of love or protection, he replied: "Yes. My way of asking for help is I contact my higher self, as long as I'm not resisting the natural way of being. I don't limit my love to anybody or anything. I see their light." Ryan went on to say, "I'm at level three Reiki now – incorporating it into daily life. I don't care about the opinions of others. I don't have any say in their beliefs. Where they're at on their journey is their business. I respect all religions. For example, I'll use any religious symbol people are comfortable with in Reiki treatments. Everybody is One in the field of Love. I like the saying, 'Everybody smiles in the same language.'"

Ryan's New Realizations

Exploring his spiritual experiences, he offered some of his new realizations. "What I think is we have a contract. The fire and burns have taken me to a happy place where I'm meant to be. There is no limit on age regarding spiritual growth. The element of fire is related to spirit and now I feel I'm going down a spiritual path. Awakening comes in all forms and in many ways. I believe we incarnate to learn lessons we couldn't learn in spirit form. Not being resistant to anything is key. Ignorance is the deepest poison – it is the main resistance. I'll help anybody who needs it, when they are ready for it."

As you can see, Ryan has undergone a spiritual transformation since the fire, but is also a work in progress. Ryan added, "I always know what's best for me, and if not, I go inside, inquiring within a contemplation/meditation. With any 'dis-ease' I'll use Reiki."

When it comes to the emotional level, Ryan says, "I've come to see it for what it is. I'm not bound by this physical body. These negative emotions are not relevant. Mind is always searching for physical items to fill it – old beliefs and thought patterns. The ego mind is resistance to flow. But the ego is something we are always going to be working on – to be forgiving and accepting of other people. There will always be unnecessary emotions. Kindness settled in for me when I realized we are all One. I'll speak up if I see an unkindness."

I asked Ryan what he feels he has learned since his encounter with fire. First, he offered, "My injury was an awakening for me. I see a lot of changes in myself. I'm emotionally a lot more stable today. Spiritually, I'm not going to say anything... it would be limited by words. I'll help anyone with a spiritual issue or a question. My favourite expression these days is: 'It's not as hard as you think.' This is what I tell people. Friends come to me and I give good advice by stepping out of the mud of the situation and seeing the bigger picture. If people make fun of me, I see it for what it is. I've moved from material values to spiritual values now and this has brought a big shift in perceptions and awareness."

Three Inspiring Messages

The biggest realizations for Ryan have come at an incredibly young age for him. He told me his most recent discovery is, "We are all One. I was told this, but I now know this to be true. It was mental before, but through experiences, I know. Everything is life-force energy – it is Love. Source energy, the Divine, that's what we are. Whatever sport you are playing, we are all on the same field."

Ryan's second realization is: "Everything is perfect as it is."

His third awakening is: "Everything is changing. Resistance to change is disharmonious, and this translates itself into disease." Ryan talked again about his love for Reiki: "I love working with Reiki. It works on all four levels of existence. The patient does the healing; Reiki supplies the patient with what's in their highest and best interest."

I asked Ryan what he would say to readers of this book - if he could offer any words of advice. "Love," he said. "I was so damaged and yet I met my highest excitement and love when that tube came out of my throat. There was no limit to the feeling of this love flowing through me. The Source (God) is Love, Peace, and cycling it through. With the experiences I've had, I can hardly define it in words – it's so intimate and natural. I like the statement, 'Silence is the language of the Gods and everything else is just a bad translation.'"

Ryan's approach to his condition is a wonderful example of what you believe, you can achieve.

∞

Exploring Thoughts, Beliefs and Attitudes

The challenges we face in life including the areas of relationships, finances, work, and health are all opportunities for our greater unfoldment. What is most important for our lesson plan in this lifetime is how we deal with our difficulties as much as the solution. It's a combination of the process plus the end result.

We have discussed our emotions and their effect on health. Now let's further explore the effects our thoughts, beliefs, attitudes and predispositions can have on our well-being.

I believe we create every so-called illness in our body. The body, like everything else in life, is a mirror of our inner thoughts and beliefs. The body is always talking to us, if we will only take the time to listen. Every cell within your body responds to every single thought you think and every word you speak.

Louise Hay, You Can Heal Your Life

Changing Our Thought Patterns

Our thoughts and beliefs are such a part of us that we usually can't see how these Mental Body patterns can affect our health and wellness. But there can be a direct relationship. A thought pattern that we have grown up with may no longer be serving our personal growth today. We may be too rigid in our beliefs and we need to open up to new ideas and possibilities as part of our journey. Maybe we need to tackle our challenges in a different way that is calling for a change in how we think, what we believe, and our attitude toward something. Perhaps we are not charitable and we need to learn to be more giving. For example, a present attitude of not giving hand-outs to beggars may have to change to learn this lesson about charity. My husband had this experience about ten years ago when he felt the urge to assist street people on his daily inner city walks. One day he even took a man shopping for lunch at small local grocers and shops so he could see how to buy the most nutrition with a small amount of money. By assisting people on the edge through his small cash gifts and personal chats, looking back on these experiences he could see that he had become more compassionate, more open to life and less closed off to the circumstances of others.

Perhaps we need to be more open to spirituality in our life and so our current focus on the material things of life needs to shift. Or possibly one needs to see the challenges of others in a new light, and a greater empathy and respect is being called for by our inner Self, Soul. Our attitudes need to shift, moderate, or purify as we make progress on our personal path, our spiritual life-journey.

If in the last few years you haven't discarded a major opinion or acquired a new one, check your pulse. You may be dead.
Gelett Burgess, author and humorist

My Mind-Body Journey

$\mathcal{I}$ have suffered from a stiff neck for about fifteen years. It's at the level of an annoyance, an inconvenience in my life, but I know that it's trying to teach me something. My stiffness often moves from my neck up into the skull from my upper trapezius muscles and my degree of discomfort relates to my physical activities such as golf and other sports. I've learned how to manage the discomfort through massage techniques using my Muscle & Joint Relief aromatherapy roll-on blend and myofascial release I do with a small hard rubber ball. Up to his point in life it was a condition I was "living with."

Uncovering Limiting Beliefs

Then one day my husband asked me if I would consent to an interview for a book he was writing. In our conversation as we delved a little deeper into the issue I began to feel that my neck was representative of inflexibility to some degree in my attitude, perhaps reflecting limiting beliefs about my abilities and career. "Maybe I'm not trusting, having faith in myself – faith in surrendering and moving forward with growing my business," I told him. "It feels like I'm sitting on the fence. I want to bring abundance into my life. I know I can earn good money but I feel like I'm sitting on the fence in a comfortable position in not venturing out, not taking any risks."

As this interview/therapy continued, I was pulling other realizations out of myself. What then emerged was, "My concern is what my life will look like if I take a risk? I'm afraid I'll not have enough spare time." A hidden fear seemed to be holding me back.

When he asked me about other insights I may have had I remembered a dream that had stayed with me for some time. In the dream which I felt was a scene from a past life, I was a man with a lot of power. I would travel around from village to village with a cadre of supporters cutting off heads for really no reason. As he (I) did this he felt proud and powerful, garnering support from his supporters. I began to relate my neck issues today with this past life. I could see that I'm experiencing neck issues to burn off karma from this past. But I also began to connect some other dots in our conversation as well; that having power in business in this life is related to my miss-use of power in the past. I've realized today that I don't want to go down that road again for fear of appearing too powerful. It dawned on me as we chatted that perhaps a fear of miss-using my power is at the core of this neck issue too?

Acknowledging My Beliefs

When our conversation circled back to my fear of not having spare time, I realized that when I'm working on my new business, I feel joyful. It is not eating up my free time. I realized that this is how I want to spend my time!

I realized my stiff neck was teaching me two lessons:

1) I don't have to be afraid of losing my free time as long as I'm doing what I love to do and I am joyful about it and not feeling resentful;

2) There is a karmic part of this too – I want to be financially successful without letting my ego take over. The power issue seems to be about being mouse-like versus being humble. I needed to find a new balance.

∞

Making Better Choices

To move forward, making better choices (being more discriminating) in thoughts, words, and deeds ask yourself:

> Am I in balance in giving and receiving love?

> Am I honoring myself as Soul?

Impatience and Healing

Impatience is another major theme in healing. Time heals all things, they say. And it is true. Impatience is a mild form of anger, of resistance to the natural flow of life. Impatience is saying, I want this to happen on my schedule, not yours or not Spirit's. Impatience leads to irritation and annoyance and can escalate upwards from there into other forms of anger.

Impatience and its other recognizable forms like "being bothered", "taking umbrage", and "quarrelsomeness" can scatter the concentration of the mind, and in the form of expressed anger creates confusion and trouble.

Slowing down and recognizing the hand of Spirit in all things is a major theme with many people. Letting go and letting God! There is a need to recognize here that there is an overall plan, a spiritual agenda to life, so we need to slow down and accept the pace that Spirit is providing us.

Walking and driving can be two very useful metaphors for us. Driving the speed limit and slowing our walking pace in the office or outdoors can help us smell the roses on our journey and make our travel time as important as our arrivals and departures.

Moving from Impatience into Tolerance and Forgiveness

To move toward greater tolerance and the ability to forgive easily, ask yourself:

> Why is my way the best way?

> What can I learn from difficult situations or events, and other people?

Greed and the Mental Body

When greed, excess and over indulgence manifest in the Mental Body, it clouds the mind to the higher values of life. It hardens the consciousness and can result in behaviours such as hypocrisy, perjury and bribery to name a few. Greed is an extreme form of selfishness and can cause illness in those that need to purify and become more giving, sharing of their time, talents, finances and possessions. As we move along this road of personal change and growth, the subtleties of giving will present themselves as opportunities to give greater service to all life.

As part of any feeling of ill health, ask yourself, where or to whom can you give more of yourself? For example, this is an excellent counterbalance to the disharmony felt in depression. When one gives from the heart with no strings attached, the extreme focus that the depressed person typically has on themselves can lift, and they can shift into a more balanced state.

Moving Into a Consciousness of Service

To shift to a greater consciousness of giving, service and contentment, you can ask yourself:

> Where can I be of greater service or be more helpful to others in my life?
>
> Can I be content with what I have?
>
> Will I be OK without?

A Hidden Side of Greed

Greed can also be present as dissatisfaction or disappointment, and if this state is allowed to manifest too often, it can result in a general unhappiness with life: there is no lasting appreciation or acceptance of what one has. This general state of unhappiness can then devolve into anxiety. Are you content with what you receive in life, or are you always seeking more? More money, recognition, time, fun and attention, are some of the ways this can be present. In this state of constantly living with the feeling of less, one is unable to feel lasting enjoyment. The antidote is gratitude and appreciation.

Creating a Consciousness of Contentment

To move into a greater feeling of contentment of being, ask yourself:

> What am I grateful for today?
>
> How can I lift others up with my positive acceptance of the way things are?
>
> In what area of my life can I love myself more?
>
> How can I grant myself forgiveness and tolerance?

The Subtle Effects of Vanity

Vanity rears its head in very subtle ways such as in the form of desiring public honours and publicity. This is the opposite of humility, a state that Soul is seeking on its human journey. An exaggerated I-ness of the mind can cloud one from their ability to listen to others and to one's inner guidance as well. Soul may need to "speak" to one in more direct ways through contemplation or other spiritual practices like yoga or walking, and if it is not being heard, changes may be required. These changes may be forced upon the physical body as a state of illness, causing one to go deeper inside to solve a challenge. In other words, the pathway to true healing in this situation may only be found in contemplation or by tuning in to other spiritual signs, as the healing methods Spirit suggests may defy the logic of the mind. As one begins to trust their inner guidance more, they move closer to humility and the acceptance of Spirit in their lives.

Another subtle aspect of vanity is shame. It springs from feelings of inadequacy, sometimes perceived as not meeting the expectations of others. It can result in an overemphasis on correctness or decorum. I am reminded of a golfer who was fortunate to be playing with a top ranked PGA Professional one day. However, every time the golfer made a bad shot he would swear. After a couple of holes of enduring this display, the Pro turned to him and said, "You know, you're not that good to be getting this upset." The golfer needed to accept his playing ability for what is was.

Cultivating Greater Humility

To move toward greater humility in interacting with others, ask yourself:

> Can I listen to others without having to add my opinion(s)?

> What makes me feel I'm better?

Attachments to the Old Way of Being

Elements of attachment can also play a strong role in our healing process. Being attached to behaviours, being locked into beliefs, having destructive attitudes, may all have to be shattered in your personal process leading to optimum wellness.

Flexibility is the virtue that Soul is craving. It needs one to be open, accommodating and a willing participant with life. Accepting change is wrapped up in this process of gaining flexibility. Your life's journey may take it into realms you have never conceived before and a thought pattern may have to be modified or eliminated along the way. Resistance can mean pain. Or the opposite is also true: pain is resistance to change. (Ryan mentioned this awakening for him.)

Where is the change required to remove the pain? Headaches are a great example of thought patterns that are no longer serving us. Migraines are a deeper manifestation, meaning that much more is on the change table that needs to be discovered, then altered in our life.

Attachment likes *respectability*, another false value that may need modification at some point. As we shift our perspective to a higher viewpoint, we realize that we need to feel comfortable in our own skin, in our self-created conditions and lifestyle. After all, we are unique beings on our own personal path of learning. Again flexibility, fluidity, the ability to go with the flow is what we are learning.

Procrastination, not letting go, hanging on to the old conditions can also cause problems that emanate from the Mental Body. So the ability to get on with things is essential. Hanging on to our comfortable situation can manifest in a form of rigidity in the body such as arthritis, or joint problems etc.

Becoming More Flexible

For letting go and moving toward more flexibility, ask yourself:

> Where can I be more flexible in my life?

> What can I let go of? If I let go, how will I benefit?

The Mind-Body can sure have its effects on our physical body and our overall harmony or vibration. As the subtle aches and issues arrive, it is our cue to go searching, to look for where the cause or causes may lie. My own discoveries about how my thought patterns contributed to my neck pain have led to other beneficial career changes, bringing more joy into my work in the process of letting go.

Yoga teaches that emotional reactions and habitual thought patterns are interconnected with habits of breathing. Breathing practices from mind-body modalities such as yoga, tai chi and Pilates can have a powerful effect by breaking through belief systems that hold you back from expressing your true potential.

Michele Hebert, Idea Fitness Journal, May 2014

The Law of Attraction (Law of Attitudes)

Thoughts are very powerful things. What you think, you become. Every thought forms into a future condition. This is why negative thoughts can be very destructive to the body and to your health. These thoughts may be subtle, so much a part of your make-up, you haven't even noticed them.

Negative thoughts are interpreted by your being in the opposite way than you would expect, and so understanding the Law of Attraction (sometimes called the Law of Attitudes) is vital to your health and well-being. When you say to yourself, "I don't want to be fat" what your mind carries as a picture is, "I want to be fat." You are left with the residual image of the negative aspects of that statement in your mind to manifest. When you say, "I don't want to get Cancer," the picture you carry is, "I want to get Cancer." Using negative terms of reference can be very damaging to your health! When we create a picture in our minds, these thought vibrations will eventually manifest and the picture comes into visibility in our lives. So, to attract health, you need to be positive about your health. You need to create positive images that can manifest.

Negative thoughts have to go. You need to find a new vocabulary that defines your world in positive terms. You want to be fit, healthy and vibrant, so the negative descriptions need to be abandoned. This means, that what you wish for becomes a positive postulate in your life. State **what you want**, not what you don't want. This is how the

Law of Attraction works. What you say about yourself becomes an image, a picture in your mind, so fill your mind with positive images that can be developed. Know that every thought you have, manifests into a future condition. You are creating your future in your present thoughts.

As DNA research has recently proved, you can literally alter your DNA's genetic setting and behavior within a matter of a moment. Your DNA listens to every word you utter to yourself, and it feels every emotion you experience. Moreover, it responds to all of them. You program yourself every second of the day, consciously and unconsciously. If you choose to, you can rewrite the program in any way you want to, provided you are truly self-aware.

Andreas Moritz, Cancer is Not a Disease, It's a Survival Mechanism

Actions are also vital. As like attracts like, to get love, you need to give love. To get respect, you need to give respect. To have a harmonious life, you have to be a force for harmony. Positive images and actions manifest as positive results.

Working with the Law of Attraction

Develop a statement about yourself that reflects three or four key positive qualities you wish to be and start the statement with "I am." Notice that this is in the present tense.

Here are three examples:

I am happy, healthy, content and creative.

I am free, wise, successful and loving.

I am confident, vibrant, and relaxed.

Once you have developed your positive statement, write this statement out fifteen times each day. This will set in motion great changes in your life, building powerful images to manifest in your life. My favourite is: *I am healthy, wise, happy and free.*

Becoming a More Positive Person

On your chosen day, resolve to think and speak <u>only</u> positive thoughts. Support the ideas of others with positive comments and suggestions – nothing negative. This practice will shift your vibration and lift you into new realms of being. You will become a positive force in the lives of others as well, just by your example.

Stress, the Silent Killer

In today's fast-paced world, we have become accustomed to stress. It's simply a part of life in Western countries. Some people actually create stress to feel like they are accomplishing a degree of success. As an example I've heard that some doctors load up their schedules for this reason. Working long hours in business can also be a badge of honor, and the busier one is, the more the ego is fed.

Movement into challenging or unknown conditions also brings stress. Originally the word was created by Hans Selye to mean 'change.' Whatever the cause of stress, we now know how destructive it can be on health. Stress can creep into our life and build up very subtly, so inconspicuously in fact that we don't even know it is there, or we simply aren't aware of its presence. But it is creating disharmonies and imbalances in our bodies that can manifest as overt health conditions. Stress from my point-of-view is about 'my will be done.' It is mind over heart, pushing the envelope so to speak. We are driven to succeed, to accomplish, to earn, to not fail, to be better, to accumulate and much more. We need to take a step back and pause. What is life all about? Is it about the things of life, or the qualities of life? Which is it for you? Have you been caught up in the pace of life? Remember, you are different from the crowd. You need to be looking at your life in your own way, through your own lenses, not through the lenses of other's expectations. Perhaps it's time to set your own agenda and pace?

Letting go is key, as well as slowing down. What would happen if you worked more creatively as opposed to trying to produce a volume of work? Slowing down enables one to work from a higher viewpoint. This is the source of great ideas, inspiration, and intuitiveness. Which is better; the power of a big idea, a wonderful insight, or high work production? Maybe knowing that you want to transition to being a more creative being will give you the incentive to make changes and reduce your stress. Creativity cannot flourish in a stressful environment. Modern companies have now incorporated gathering places into their work environments for collaboration and to help staff de-stress and laugh a little. Others have included fitness and sports facilities for the same purpose. Some have even built contemplation, meditation and prayer rooms for their people, a strong indication of the awareness that poor staff health, absenteeism and lower productivity can result from stress. I have several corporate clients that bring me into their offices to offer chair massages to their staff.

So how can you make changes? Visualization in contemplation can be a big aid to reducing stress, reducing the impact on one's immune and cardiovascular systems. I'm certain that the high incidence of heart attack in our society is in part related to suppressing the heartfelt desires of the higher Self, Soul. Stress hormones can also have a very negative effect on joints and the spine.

Reducing Stress in Your Life.

One sure way to reduce stress in your life - with everyone you meet in your day, give them more of your time and a smile. Treat them like part of your extended family and enjoy the moments together. Unconditional love is diminishing in our fast-paced world, so bring it back with your new expanded meaning of family to include everyone in your wide circle of relationships as family.

At the same time, make a conscious effort to slow your pace of walking and driving. Count your travel time as important time, not just transit time. Make it a time to muse, contemplate, and decompress. Leave for meetings and appointments ahead of schedule so you have plenty of time to chill before your connection. It is much healthier living in a relaxed manner. If you need to, to accomplish this, take something out of your day to make room for your new pace. If you are rushing, you will never have time to give to your new "family" at every turn in your day.

Making Health-Conscious Choices: Thoughts, Words and Beliefs

On each line, I invite you to note where you can take a new step into greater harmony along your path to optimum health.

Negative State	A Step I Can Take	Conscious Choice
Impatience		**Patience**
Being Bothered, Quarrelsomeness		Letting Go, Slowing Down
Intolerance		**Forgiveness, Tolerance,**
I Am Right		Accepting of others
Greed, Selfishness		**Giving, Sharing**
Dissatisfaction		No-strings-attached Giving
Unhappiness with Life		Contentment
Always Seeking More		Gratitude, Appreciation
Vanity		**Humility**

Shame, Inadequacy	Listening to Others
Correctness, Decorum, Respectability	Confidence, Relaxed
Attachments	**Flexibility**
Resistance to Change	Going With the Flow
Procrastination	Get it Done
Negative Thoughts	**Positive Outlook**
Bringing Others Down	Lifting Others Up
Depressing, A Downer	Happiness
Disagreeing with Others	Supporting Others
Stress in Your Life	**Relaxed**
Work Production is Valued	Creativity is Valued
Fast pace	Slowing Down-Creative Pace
Rushing into the Future	Living in the Moment

But regardless of what supplements you take and what kind of exercise you do, when all is said and done it is your attitude, your beliefs, and your daily thought patterns that have the most profound effect on your health.

Cristiane Northrup, MD, The Wisdom of Menopause

6

Create Your Life Anew –
Making Conscious Choices

Every time you find yourself judging or criticizing, no matter how small, remind yourself that what goes out comes back. You may want to stop limiting your possibilities and change your thinking to something wonderful.

Louise Hay, The Power is Within You

What comes around, goes around, is another way of describing karma. What we say, do, how we react, treat others, what we put in or on our bodies all returns to us in the form of a lesson – karma. Much of the time, these lessons return to us as health challenges, opportunities to learn and grow. Karma teaches us to make better, more conscious, enlightened choices.

Let's take a look at Rebecca's experience, what turned out to be a major life lesson for her.

Rebecca's Story

*R*ebecca's world was rocked one day when she returned home from work to find her husband dead. He had died shortly after she had left for work and had been laying there on the floor all day. They had only been married three years. Her life, however, was about to take another awful turn. At the funeral she was asked by friends, "Who is that lady bawling over there?" A little later, the woman approached Rebecca and was very angry with her and it was in that moment Rebecca realized this woman had a romantic connection with her husband! Soon it became apparent her husband had been having an affair throughout their marriage. Rebecca's life hit bottom. First a tragic loss, then a betrayal. Rebecca later determined her husband could not face leaving her and had a heart attack.

As time went on, Rebecca found that she was the only one who didn't know about the affair. The whole family knew! "I could not tell him what a S.O.B. he was now that he was dead. I could not face this situation. I was really hurt because I trusted him," she confided. "But I knew deep down I had caused this. I used to go out with married men in my younger days. I liked married men because they were safe. One even arrived on my doorstep with his suitcase after leaving his wife. I had to send him home. Now it was payback time."

A Sore Throat – Holding it In

It still didn't make Rebecca's life any easier knowing she had to take responsibility for her husband's betrayal. As time went on, her throat became sore. "It was very hoarse," she recounted. "I finally made an appointment with my doctor six months later. On examination he could find nothing wrong. He had me sit down and asked me, 'What's been happening these last six months?' I broke down in a flood of tears and cried and cried. I told him the whole story. I had been holding back, not expressing myself – all of my sadness, disappointment and hurt. I had no one I could share this with. I couldn't talk about it at work, I had no family at the time and my one close friend was away. I was alone.

"I felt the crying was the start of a healing, getting it out of my system. The doctor didn't give me anything for my throat but he did prescribe an antidepressant. I took a quarter pill a day for two weeks. My throat began to heal and within two weeks it was better. Soon after that I found my current spiritual path which confirmed my thoughts about karma and reincarnation.

Help from Contemplation and Dreams

"Dreams also played a part in my spiritual growth during my healing time following the death and betrayal. One night I had a dream of a beautiful large white wolf. He was standing up on a bluff. I thought he was going to attack me, but instead he attacked the dark side of me, protecting me. It was a spiritual awakening for me." It was at this point Rebecca revealed she was a recovering alcoholic. She had gained sobriety about a year before her husband's death after a friend had introduced her to Alcoholics Anonymous. "The dream was telling me to be careful. It helped me to see how easily I could slip back. It wouldn't take much. I tend to write my dreams in cycles. If I don't journal, a dream will come up that I need to write down, and this pulls me back into journaling.

"After finding my new spiritual path, I felt love. I was on a spiritual high. I had a sense of belonging now. It's the family I never had. This helped me to move past my experiences, the betrayal and anger, and I was able to move forward and let go. I knew it was karma but the contemplations I started to practice were the key to moving on. Today, Spirit is such a part of my life and I see it at work in my life all the time now.

"Contemplation is now a tool I use all the time. As a child I would talk to my guardian angel, so contemplation was a natural progression for me. I ask God for help when I need it, but I know I have to help myself first, to have the willingness to do better, to be better. So asking is also a part of my being today. The way it works best for me is gratefulness – to be connected to the higher power."

Shaped by the Past

Rebecca also told me about her upbringing which has had a great influence on her life. Her mother was a poor immigrant that could not afford children. Her mother told her she would try to abort her pregnancies, but Rebecca was born in spite of this. Rebecca would reply to her mother, "I was meant to be."

"I've had to keep a lot inside in my life like watching my mother get beaten and even being beaten myself as a child. I could tell no one. This builds up. The walls build up. I was afraid to express myself."

At age twenty-six, Rebecca was bulimic and in a marriage she had to leave. She began drinking to numb the pain, yet she associated alcohol with fun. It was an escape for her. She carried her drinking into the second marriage, and as she began to feel something was wrong, her drinking increased.

Rebecca continued, "My friend talked me into going to AA when I was ready to face the disease and life around me. When my world fell apart, I resisted alcohol in spite of everything that happened. AA is a spiritual program and connected me with the higher power. It was a stepping stone to my spiritual path today. AA helped me let go of the emotions. I have so much trust in Spirit now. Life has become so much easier, with my daily contemplations which give me my spiritual strength. But I have to continually work at it – to deal with the betrayal, and the alcohol.

"I don't want to go back to where I was. I can't slack off. I want to live every day with gratefulness. I am so happy to be healthy, alive and sober, to be connected to a higher power.

Discovering My Life Mission

"I realize now why I'm here. I have a mission. The little I do helps others. By sharing our experiences, this also helps others. I've discovered I need to let go of the past and live in the present moment. In my experience burning off karma, I got a taste of my own medicine. I felt safe with married men. I never meant to hurt anyone but I still had to pay for this - it was selfish. I was just thinking of myself. With my husband's death and betrayal it all came to a head. It was interesting that day: his sons were working around his house all day and never knew he was dead inside. I was the one who was meant to find him. I needed to have the full effect of that experience.

The Throat Metaphor

"Today my throat acts up from time to time but I've discovered that if I don't get my feelings off my chest, it returns, particularly if I'm tired, stressed or sad. For example, if I start housework and my voice starts changing, I know it's time to quit. If I talk my feelings out, my throat returns to normal. My present husband today is a "controller" and so he is my teacher in this respect. My throat comes on unexpectedly and leaves as quickly when I express my feelings.

"My daily contemplations have been a big help in me working with my throat 'messages.' If I sit quietly, I'll have an inner connection. It relaxes me and makes a difference in the hoarseness. It calms my voice and my being. My throat is like a barometer telling me to speak up, slow down, and smarten up. All the time I'm getting this guidance."

∞

Karma – Why We are Here

Karma is the cause of our current family setting, other relationships, friends, work, country, financial circumstances, genetic predispositions, personal preferences, character and wellness. These components of our life are a precisely constructed lesson package.

The set of circumstances we call our life is a bundle of karma that has been shaped by our past thoughts, words and actions. These karmic influences come from our past lives as Soul, and this present lifetime as well, and attract us to people, places and things, all for our greater unfoldment. As an example, falling in love is really falling into karma - i.e. a karmic attraction. The issues that need the most attention are brought to us in our closest relationships - spouses, family, friends and work associates. We are attracted to these people, conditions and situations which can also be referred to as karmic attraction.

Our karma (our lessons in this life) has been earned and what we call the good in our lives can be attributed to our good acts of previous times. And the so called bad in our lives, our challenges, can be traced to our past as well, areas of needed growth today. Karma is usually rebalanced and resolved through three avenues: financial, service and pain. Of the three, it seems that pain and discomfort move us forward the most and reshape us into a better version of who we are.

Disharmonies occur in our bodies for our purification from outmoded physical, mental, and emotional habits, and patterns from our past. As discussed before, these disharmonies can manifest in the body as discomfort, chronic conditions, illness, disease and even accidents and injury. These patterns can stem from genetic influences which have been shaped by our past thoughts words and deeds and result in our emotional make-up, attitudes, thought patterns and predispositions today.

An integral part of the healing process is taking responsibility, and so karma can be part of our current health – our well-being. Karmic patterns can be the sole cause of an imbalance or simply a part of it. Let's now take a look at what Anastasia has been dealing with.

Anastasia's Story

*A*nastasia has been living with back pain, what she calls her "rotten back" for over sixty years. She was working at age seventeen when she twisted it, and since that time has been living with back pain on and off all her life. "It's been more on than off," she told me, "and I've been seeing chiropractors for years."

In 1987 I even saw a Shaman. He went into contemplation, and when he came out he told me he could take the edge off it, but nothing more. "Over the years," Anastasia told me, "when I have to do something, make a change in life, and when I resist, my back goes out. Then I need to see a chiropractor. For example, when I needed to leave the big city to help my mom in a town a few hours away, I resisted and got a bad back again. When I needed to move again, and resisted, I fell and broke my hip! This is a pattern of not listening and not following through, not catching on to what I need to do," she told me.

Contemplations Lead to Acceptance

Anastasia continued: "Through daily contemplations, morning and before bedtime, I have grown into a kind of acceptance. This acceptance has been aided by about fifteen powerful and clear dreams that have given me a look at past lives where this bad back issue all began. These experiences were so very clear and I knew it was me doing these terrible things – Oh my God! I needed to see them and accept their realities. And so certain people were in my life this time again.

"This has been a real gift. I can see the causes of my bad back now – karma. Looking back in this present life I know where I've gone wrong. I've seen in these dreams where I was a victim, but, I can extrapolate now what I did as the cause factors. In many of these lives, I was with people I've met and interacted with in this life. I now know what I did and the results of my past actions. I've learned a few things - like I need to learn to listen.

"I have a strong feeling I have to live with this condition. In other words, I need to pay off this karma. After sixty years, I've come to a point of acceptance now that I need to go through it. I'm not sure if I should be looking for a healing because it won't fix the cause which I earned. I need to wear it.

I know I'm Protected

"Looking back on my life, I can see that I've been protected. I've been prevented from doing stupid things, and kept out of harm's way. For example, one night I was volunteering and a friend came in and talked to me way past closing time, delaying my normal time of departure. On the way home I passed two serious accidents within two blocks. I just knew I was protected from that experience. Also I've had pneumonia eight times. On one occasion I was out for four days, it was so serious. So I'm being protected and I also know that there is no way I'm going to get out of this life until I'm done, until I've burned off my karma. So I get help when I need it, but I also need to pay. All in all, I've had a good life in spite of this awful back, so I just need to find the balance.

Moving Away from Anger

"I've had a temper all my life, but I could control it if the circumstances were not terribly personal. Today, I've come along way. I let it be, now. I see others as just what they are, Souls with a

114

lot to learn. This makes it easier to let go of situations and to let the anger go with it.

"I know I can't fight my back situation. I just go to the chiropractor if I need to. It gets fixed for a week or so. I know I have to go through a number of things at this point. Right now it's so bad I can hardly walk and I'm using a walker instead of a cane. I know I have to see a surgeon about surgery. It's that or a nursing home.

"But my constitution is strong after thirty-five years on my spiritual journey. It's been my faith that has kept me on my feet, learning to cope with the pain. I don't say: 'Why me?' It's fine if this is the way it works. I know whatever happens, happens for a reason. And I've learned a few things along the way, particularly about karma. After all these years, there has had to be some cleansing going on with me. I've seen fifteen past lives but there is much more to clean up. My past life dream experiences connected me to people I've met in this life such as my father and other relationships. I've met one person in this life that I was married to several times in the past, but I was forced into it by my father on those occasions. I hope I've said good bye to those sets of circumstances now.

Detachment, another Key

"Key for me in my spiritual growth in this life has been learning more about detachment. Some things bothered me for years, and if I can say no to these things – to let go – I'm better off. These things include stuff and people I need to let be. They have to live their life. So I'm detaching myself from things that don't mean anything anymore. When you see the past so clearly, you know it's a fact. I needed to come into agreement with it, acknowledge it and let it go. Memories are not good for me. I need to let it go and focus on the present.

"For me, my dreams reinforced the reality of reincarnation and that things from the past have to be dealt with. Some people don't see this, and repeat it over and over again. I want to finish it off, whatever I can, not incurring any more karma in these relationships forever."

∞

A Path to Resolving Karma

First, as part of our personal search for truth and rebalancing, we need to understand that karma is playing a primary role in our current overall set of conditions and is the reason why we are having this human experience. If we had no karma, there would be no need for being here. Our growth would be finished here in this big schoolhouse and we would be graduated to a "college" or "university" for Soul's greater purification in a higher realm, another spiritual plane, universe or heaven. So everyone has karma to recognize, deal with and learn from.

One needs to take responsibility for it. At this point you may not understand what it is, but you need to be willing to accept that if there is a health problem, karma could be involved in some way. This means you are open to seeking the underlying cause or causes that were set in motion in the past and to make changes in rebalancing these conditions emanating from the past. This usually entails re-evaluating emotional responses and thoughts that underlie interactions with others

You will also need to be prepared to accept the conscious realizations when you uncover them or when they are revealed to you. Like Anastasia, there is the possibility that you were quite an awful person in a past setting, and you need to be able to see this, accept it for what it was, and then see how it fits with your present circumstances.

You need to find ways to resolve the pattern that is no longer serving you. At this juncture there are some big keys to moving forward; acceptance of the truth about your past, and forgiveness and apologizing to those you hurt (remember Therese). This process is about changing. It involves shifting to a new space, a new consciousness of being.

Changes of any magnitude seem to only work with major incentives whether they are negative or positive, to move out of our physical, emotional and mental comfort zones. Tilting the scales from greed to giving, from anger to forgiveness, from ego to humility or from lying and cheating to total honesty can be a lifetime project for us, or can occur in a moment, an epiphany. Some people have lifetimes filled with change and progress, and others seem to have very predictable linear lifetimes, growing in a very stable setting or set of conditions. Again, the caution here is not to judge your life by what you see in others.

Healing from Past Life influences

As with examining the physical and emotional bodies, like Anastasia, you need to be the active participant in designing your own path to wholeness when it comes to resolving karmic issues.

Contemplation or meditation in the form of creative visualization is one key, and in combination with singing/chanting HU or another spiritually charged sound like OM, can work wonders to help you resolve your karma. In contemplation you can see yourself in a more detached way on the stage of life and previously invisible patterns can be made visible. Make this a regular good habit, a part of your day that you dedicate to yourself and the changes that you would like to happen in your life. I've included more on contemplation as a tool to develop your inner guidance in a later chapter.

Never be afraid to sit awhile and think.

Lorraine Hansberry, *A Raisin in the Sun*

Karen's Story

Karen found herself in a condition without explanation, a severely impaired neck and shoulder. She was in tremendous pain with seemingly no cause. The condition just showed up one day. She tried her regular doctor who prescribed pain medicine and muscle relaxants. These worked a little for a day or two but she was still off work, quite paralyzed by the condition.

The next week she was in to see her doctor for another visit and he admitted he was stumped about her condition. He could not find anything that could be the visible cause or trigger. He gave her a reference to a specialist in the local hospital, but also advised that because this specialist was the best in the country, he was in great demand and that it may take months to be able to see him. She left feeling quite bewildered but on arriving home, called to set up an appointment. Her doctor had already called to make the referral but the specialist's assistant did not seem optimistic about an early visit.

Shortly thereafter, she got a call back. Could she come in tomorrow? This was astonishing but what was even more amazing was that when she met the doctor, they realized they knew each other. They used to work together years ago when he was putting himself through medical school.

Within a few days of the visit and his treatment, she was back to normal! In a subsequent contemplation she realized there was some lingering karma between them that needed to be smoothed over. Her neck and shoulder condition was a gift from Spirit to bring her together with the specialist once again in this lifetime to resolve the issue forever.

∞

Healing yourself is connected to healing others.

Yoko Ono, artist, musician and author

Addressing Personal Karma

If your challenge(s) today involve another person(s), you can try a contemplation. After a few minutes of relaxation, visualize meeting the person as Soul. Be kind and open with the person and have a conversation with them. Start with pleasantries and then move the conversation to the subject of your problems. Explain your side, then listen for them to explain their viewpoint.

Be open. Don't judge them. Ask them how you can heal the situation and move forward.

This technique can have dramatic results and open your eyes to another viewpoint.

Conscious Choices - Keys to Resolving Health Karma

1   Asking for help: Ask Spirit, God, a religious figure or your spiritual guide to help you see what past thoughts words and deeds may be playing a part in your present situation.

2   Listen and look for answers: These may come in the form of dreams, Signs, a book or story, a flash of insight and more.

3   Service to others: Selfless giving is another key to successfully unravelling a challenge. This takes the attention off the self and places it outward on others. It has the effect of opening the heart which is the gateway to Soul and to Spirit. With a genuinely open heart, the love of God enters and has an opportunity to impress upon your being the steps you need to take regain good health. This may include a conscious realization of what needs to change within you. It could also provide you with a direct perception of the past circumstances and behaviours that set your present life conditions in motion so that you can begin to make changes. It could also open you up to greater receptivity and to new alternatives you have never considered before.

4   Charity: Generosity also opens the heart. Being generous with your time, talents and money is a great way to make changes in your life and well-being. Start with what you can and go from there. Limited finances, poor mobility or a perceived lack of skill or knowledge are just forms of procrastination. Volunteering can be a large part of your charity adventure into giving. We all have opportunities to be charitable and this represents a polar opposite move forward, away from many limiting traits that we are leaving behind as we expand in consciousness.

5   Giving Love: In this context, I am talking about spiritual love. Love has many faces. For you it could mean to bring joy into the lives of others by being cheerful. Or it may be by being humorous, bringing lightness to the lives of those around you. In other ways, one can be a good listener or interact with others with a new level of respect for their ideas and beliefs by reinforcing the choices they make as opposed to commenting with your opinion. This openness has a way of reflecting inward too, helping you open up to new healing possibilities and messages from the heart that can reveal solutions to past causes.

6   Silent Acts of Service: This process of silently giving love will positively change you! Find one thing you can do each day for someone else without seeking any recognition or thanks. Do it quietly and discretely.

7   Journaling: This can be very therapeutic and open up channels of insight and intuition you never thought possible. Remember, if you are feeling resistant to this idea,   you should really do it! By recording my dreams, spiritual experiences and the events of my life, I have found I am better able to make connections and receive guidance that can help me solve problems big and small, steer clear of pitfalls plus avoid making costly mistakes. One technique is writing a letter to God. It is also a wonderful way to express your feelings and order your thoughts.

Journaling also has the benefit of allowing your thoughts to free-flow and the answers you seek can pour out onto the page.

8   **Being Grateful**: You would be amazed at how this can change your life. Begin to appreciate the wonderful people, things and circumstances of your life. This creates a positive, can-do attitude and results in a major shift in energy. It turns a negative downward spiral into a positive uplifting spiral. I suggest a daily journal entry at the end of your day that simply says, I am grateful for (a person, friends, gifts from spirit, money, work, home, new realization etc.) today. Don't be afraid to share your appreciation of others with them and build them up too. Everyone loves to be appreciated!

We can move past our karma but it does take an effort on our part. You have to be willing to explore and make changes, and possibly reinvent yourself in the process.

What is ill health? It's the result of a deliberate or else an unconscious violation of laws for a period of time. This ignorance of karmic law reflects imperfection. Healing then means doing something in a new way to regain health.

Harold Klemp, A Modern Prophet Answers Your Key Questions about Life, Book 2

7

Tapping Your Inner Guidance: Making Choices from Your Highest Perspective

We are all in a process of transformation to something greater than our current state of enlightenment....and so it is a soul's destiny to search for truth in their experiences in order to gain wisdom.

Michael Newton, Ph.D., Journey of Souls

Stella's Life-transformation

My friend Stella has a dual career as a natural health practitioner and another work assignment that involves a lot of travel. As she was about to board a flight one day, an airline staff person approached her to let her know she needed to call her family on an urgent matter. Upon talking to her brother-in-law, she heard that her mother had just died of a massive heart attack. She was in total shock. Her life was loaded up with stress as she had just purchased her first home after many years of renting, and she had yet to close on the deal. Her loss just added other burdens, having to look after the funeral arrangements as well as pack up a quarter lifetime of possessions and move. "The move was hard," she told me, "letting go of the old apartment and its memories."

Thirty days later she started to lose weight, rapidly dropping from one-hundred-and-five to eighty-eight pounds over a three week period. But she continued to work. A few more weeks down the road she started to get comments from co-workers about how gaunt she looked, yet she still resisted seeing a doctor. Finally after six months of denial about her condition, she relented and scheduled a visit. It wasn't good. Her doctor thought she might have thyroid Cancer! He referred her on to an Endocrinologist who diagnosed her condition as something quite different, Graves' disease. "There is a lot of mystery surrounding this condition as to causes and cures," he informed her, but he gave her some literature to read. The information indicated that one of the triggers for Graves' is psychological and emotional stress.

Facing Unresolved Issues

"I remember reflecting on my life at that time," Stella told me. "I realized I had not told my mother about my new condo, wanting to surprise her when I closed the deal. It felt like an unresolved issue. I had never settled down and married, had children, bought a home and become a doctor like they had hoped. I realized deep down I wanted to please my mother with this big step of settling down, but now I could not share my joy with her. I could see subconsciously I had been always trying to please my parents.

"My condition had caused my dramatic weight loss because I could not keep food down. Diarrhea was also a big part of the issue, plus I had tremors in my hands as well as heart palpitations. With all of this, my anxiety soared. The Graves' was speeding things up and I was constantly hot. I was told the condition could lead to a heart attack, but I was not paying attention, I was in denial.

"On accepting treatment, the doctor's protocol to control my metabolism involved some horrible medicine which gave me hives and skin rashes. However it worked, allowing me to regain my weight and to stop shaking. The specialist though, also wanted to give me radiation treatments to prevent Cancer from developing. But I knew it would destroy my thyroid, an important gland that controls metabolism, affecting every function of the body. I'd need to be placed on synthetic hormones for the rest of my life. I steadfastly declined the radiation, but accepted the prescription cortisone cream for the terrible skin conditions caused by the drugs.

Taking Responsibility Physically and Spiritually

"At this point in my experience I realized deep down I needed to take responsibility for my condition. I went for acupuncture and also saw a Chinese Medicine specialist who gave me some traditional Chinese herbal remedies. Moving more into the process of taking responsibility for what I was experiencing, I began to use all the spiritual responses I could muster to engage all my senses. What emerged was emotional – shock and a sense of guilt. I realized I felt like a failure not fulfilling my parent's dream. I had many talents as a child and youth including high academic aptitudes, skilled piano playing and creative writing. My parents had high expectations, yet I knew I had a different calling other than getting married, having kids and developing my current talents. But my parents being Asian held these strong traditional expectations.

"I had reinvigorated my contemplation practice and had begun to use creative visualization. One day, looking for techniques to help me heal, I read a book on spiritual guides and inner world temples, and as I scanned down a list of these inner masters, I saw the name Ori Diogo. I read his noted role: He was in charge of healing on the Astral (emotional) Plane, and his name immediately resonated with me. In my daily contemplation I began to sing his name out loud and picture myself in the spiritual healing temple working with him in the higher worlds. I'd see myself on a table singing HU, a healing sound for me, envisaging the colour orange around my throat. I could feel it and see it. I also enveloped myself in a blue light to heal my emotions.

"As time went on, I went from initially pleading and bargaining (with the thought of cancer gripping me), asking for this condition to be taken away, to accepting things for what they were - to a state of peacefulness. I was letting go and in that process I shifted and felt lifted. My contemplations and visualization exercises were now giving me gentle reassurances from the Holy Spirit. I got a strong feeling it would all work out as I let go of self-judgement.

Self-discovery Exercises

"Part of my self-discovery process involved using my writing talents. I kept a healing journal, tracking my feelings and emotions – I got it all out. For me it was a way of getting rid of it. What also helped me was an exercise, writing a special phrase fifteen times: 'I am loved.' I would express it in stanzas like a poem, a mantra. Through writing I realized I had not been expressing myself or speaking my truth! A deep seated fear of ridicule was coming from my Asian cultural background, and being female. I discovered part of my healing was learning to speak up.

"Today, I'm in remission. On my last visit to the doctor I was jumping for joy when he told me I would no longer need the drugs. However, I continue to take Chinese herbs to keep in balance and I have acupuncture treatments regularly.

"I'm continuing to find my voice and this is even finding its way into public presentations I'm doing. I'm now much more relaxed about this. I'm listening and paying attention to inner nudges. Before, I was an overachiever, addicted to perfection, so always controlled by fear of criticism. Today, I'm much more relaxed.

Healing Happens on All Levels

"I finally came to understand that healing happens on all levels (Physical, emotional, causal, mental and spiritual). I reached an acceptance of myself the way I am. What I really needed was self-acceptance. And I needed to experience this on a cellular level, not being attached to any particular outcome. I experienced a lot of growth at that time, accepting myself in my own skin. Growing up being female and Asian, a visible minority with a sensitive constitution in a Western society, I had even chosen a career involving a lot of travel and this underscored my issue of not seeming to make a commitment to being here. My parents wanted me to be a doctor but I became a holistic practitioner instead. But I burned out of that career because I would go go go. I seemed to be a Type A personality, always trying to please my clients at my own expense. I wasn't honoring myself."

Stella also told me how a dream helped her: it was a turning point in her healing journey. "I was taking a walk with my spiritual guide in the dream," she reflected. "He was asking: 'Do you understand? Do you understand?' As time went on I had to learn where this issue was coming from. It came back to accepting myself the way I am – self love. I was paying lip service to the idea up until that point. It just wasn't sinking in. Through this illness experience, it has now sunk in!"

Stella continued, "Graves' Disease turned out to be a big life-transformation for me. My healing even translated into new awakenings about my relationships – that I was addicted to dysfunctional liaisons. I realized I had chosen partners who were emotionally unavailable, and this was detrimental to my spiritual growth. Today, I'm totally free. I no longer choose involvements out of need. If I choose to be with a partner, they will also be on a spiritual journey.

Healing: It Comes Back to Love

"I can also see I've modified so that I'm not so hard on myself. I'm perfect by not being perfect. I'm accepting each moment as perfect. I'm now more authentic, yet when I speak up, it is with grace. I've now accepted as fact that I'm loved by my parents and God. I'm letting something come in instead of blocking it. This something is love. I now have an expanded awareness of it. It is love that we're here for. It all comes back to loving yourself first, then loving God, family and others."

Stella shared her final thoughts on her journey: "Always remember to come back to love. It's so simple yet so profound. Giving service is part of this love. We are here to serve others. If you embrace this in your whole being, healing can occur."

∞

The Power of Going Within

If you truly wish to solve your challenges in life, as Stella's experience shows us, you will want to go within and tap your inner guidance (intuition, insight, the creative power of Soul are other terms) to make the most conscious choices possible. There are two methods that appear to be interchangeable in leading you to a greater ability to listen within yourself, to expand your consciousness and enjoy spiritual connectedness: meditation and contemplation. However there is a difference in the methods. The meditative technique as given by Eastern teachers is practiced by sitting still and gazing into the Third Eye and viewing what may be given to the meditator. It is basically a passive approach in trying to draw awareness into oneself to attain an inner connection. This method is suited to the slower Eastern world lifestyle and can be a challenge for the Western lifestyle which is faster-paced.

Contemplation, which is what I practice every day for twenty to thirty minutes, is quite different. In this practice, one begins by sitting or lying down. The contemplation can start by closing the eyes and taking a few deep breaths to relax. Chanting a spiritual sound (such as HU or Om) to spiritualize the consciousness can help your contemplation experience although it is not necessary. In contemplation one may gently place their attention on the screen of their imagination. During this time of inward reflection, the person can look for inner spiritual light or listen for inner spiritual sounds, or visualize something like a goal. Use of the imagination is key. During contemplation, one can also focus on ideas, challenges, thoughts, or a spiritual principle etc. Some describe contemplation as a form of wondering about something. It is different from Eastern meditation in that it is an active process of inner exploration. The key is bypassing conscious thinking, getting above the mind so to speak, and accessing the soul perspective.

Contemplation is one of the greatest tools of good health I can offer you. Not only is contemplation about giving yourself personal time, an opportunity to give yourself some love, it can be an amazing opportunity to de-stress and let go of problems. It can offer you an opportunity to tune in to your inner being, gain a higher perspective on life's events and receive answers to life's challenges. It is a gentle process of going inward to connect with Soul and Spirit and is a key vehicle to access your creativity and get the direction and guidance you need. This is how to make the most conscious choices in life. You want to go the highest source, Soul. Soul (the inner you) is an integral part of the body of Spirit and so if a question can be asked, there is always an answer available. So the more proficient you are at contemplation, the better your access to intuition, insight and inner guidance.

The mind is really a tool of the human self and runs on its own learned tracks. So it can only play back its thoughts from a memory bank of its own experiences. Think of the mind as a computer and Soul as the computer operator. In solving life challenges, you will want to get above this pool of mind experiences and tap the creative power of Soul. This is the source of true innovation, insight and fresh ideas. So, creativity is going beyond the limits of the mind, and contemplation is a path I recommend in order to make choices for your highest good.

The ultimate value of life depends upon awareness and the power of contemplation rather than upon mere survival.

Aristotle

Asking for Help

A primary step in taking charge of your health is asking for help. Reflecting back on her challenge with Graves Disease, Stella sought inner direction. You must be clear with your questions so the answers you seek will be clear as well. Asking is also best done as part of a process of self-help and self-examination. That is, your best approach is to ask for assistance in solving your challenge, not to ask for your challenge to be solved for you. You need to take responsibility for your condition, after all you created it in some way and it is now present to teach you something about yourself so you can make changes. So understanding that your healing is a process of discovery and learning, your questions should be framed to facilitate this process.

Some good questions to ask are:

What do I need to learn?

What do I need to let go of that is no longer serving me?

How can I change and grow to be a better person?

How can I love more?

What do I need to bring into my life to improve it? Could this be a quality of love? (See list in the Appendix.)

Can you please help me solve this challenge in the way you see fit? (Here you are asking to be connected to information, people or other resources that can help you solve your challenge.)

These types of questions imply a partnership with Spirit. You are seeking guidance and taking responsibility for your health, rather than simply asking for a healing or general help. By taking charge, you are actually accelerating the recovery or rebalancing process. Ask yourself, How long do I want to be in this situation? What am I willing to do to move through this condition?

This process of asking penetrating/probing questions will move you out of your traditional comfort zone and into the world of total responsibility. You do everything you can do to solve your challenge.

You have to leave the city of your comfort and go into the wilderness of your intuition. What you'll discover will be wonderful. What you'll discover is yourself.

Alan Alda, Actor, Director, Screenwriter and Author

Who to Ask?

Asking for help from your highest source is a personal choice. You could direct your request to Spirit, or the Holy Spirit, or the Life Force. You may have a religious figure that you call upon for help such as Jesus or Muhammad. You may call upon God or by any name such as Allah, or there may be a spiritual guide or Master in your life that you can call upon for assistance.

Now be prepared to receive!

How to Receive Answers to Your Questions

Spirit (or Its chosen name for you as discussed above) speaks to us in many ways: dreams, signs, insights and nudges, books, and the words of others are some of the possibilities. The key is to be aware of these ways and the messages when they present themselves.

There are an infinite number of paths you can take, and your path will be unique to your need to learn and your overall lesson plan in this lifetime. Therefore, you first of all need to be open to what is presented. After all you are now asking Soul, Spirit or God for guidance, not your mind. You are reaching for answers from on high, otherwise you would have solved your issues by now with brainpower. Not that brainpower isn't useful, but the greater perception here is that you need something new and fresh to face your challenges head on. (Reminder: if you keep on doing what you're doing, you'll keep on getting what you're getting.) Also note that your need to grow spiritually is wrapped up in the search for optimum health, and so there may be multiple aspects you need to look at; emotional responses, mental thoughts, physical impediments and more that require your attention.

Keeping a Journal

As Stella mentioned it can be very beneficial to keep a journal or diary. This will allow you to record the impressions you receive in contemplations, insights you receive, and of course a record of health and fitness. You will also be recording what you feel you are learning on your personal journey. What have you realized? How have you changed lately?

It is best to make a daily entry, even if it is just one line that says how you feel today. Keep it by your bedside to also record your dreams.

Tapping the Creative Power of Soul with Yoga

We all know yoga is good for fitness but it can also be a spiritual practice and a wonderful healing companion. It opens up the body and keeps it receptive and flexible and can be an aid to detoxification. These benefits also translate to other levels of your being – your emotional, causal, and mental bodies. When something changes, opens or expands on one level, it has the effect of initiating a similar action in another part of us - as above, so below. Yoga can be excellent for balancing the energy centers (chakras), and certain postures can have specific benefits for healing and integration on all levels. Most types or brands of yoga encourage inner reflection in postures such as svasana where one is lying down, or mountain pose which is a standing posture. The breath work in some yoga styles also has the effect of helping one connect to the calm quiet place within.

Spirituality is critical in our lives, because it's not necessarily religion. It's believing in something and identifying a purpose for being, and recognizing that there's more to you than just the physical and emotional side of yourself.

Dr. Fabrizio Mancini

From an interview on his book, The Power of Self-Healing

8

Fitness –

Key to Optimum Health

Your lifestyle is the most important factor affecting your personal well-being, but most people don't know how to make the right choices to live their best life....Physical activity and exercise lead to less disease, a longer life, and enhanced quality of life.

Werner and Sharon Hoeger, authors of Fitness & Wellness

Stanley is a personal trainer friend of mine but he is also a holistic trainer too. He shared with me some of his philosophy: "For me to train, I want to be in optimum shape – I want to be more aware and have a healthy self on all levels. By doing this it gets me where I'm going with a lot less wear and tear," he said. "With me, it's becoming aware in the knowing state so you don't have to experience things in the physical state. So I eat right, I hear and sense what I'm to do on the inner dimensions – intuition, insight and knowingness are the result. This is what I like to pass on to my clients."

When I asked Stanley how this affects his client relationships, he responded, "When I start with a new client, I tell them my overall approach to training is on these four levels; physical, emotional, mental and spiritual, and that I use the HU. I let them know I sing it for many reasons and suggest they may also want to use it to help themselves. I tell them, 'It's non-denominational and connects you to your highest self.'

"When I accept a new client it's a process that unfolds over the next six months. I plant spiritual seeds. That's simply being who I am most of the time. Naturally, some clients are more open to this approach than others, and at the beginning of a new client relationship, I never know how things are going to go with my body-mind-emotions-soul program method.

"This is what makes my job so amazing. This physical self is just a coat. It's not who we are. We can be an instrument of love and self-discovery in helping people find out more of their true self. Knowing this brings joy to my life. I love it!

∞

Being an Open Channel for Spirit

What my friend Stan is doing pretty much sums up my approach to health and wellness as well. My role is to be an open channel for Spirit and to help my clients and students move forward in life. This usually involves helping them make changes on one or more levels whether they realize it or not. It can involve diet. It can mean smoothing out the emotional responses to life situations. It can mean gaining a better understanding of the principle of cause and effect – what we give out, we get back (karma), and it also includes being aware of the power of our thoughts – knowing what we think and believe, eventually takes form in our lives.

All of these body-mind-emotions-spirit elements are integral to my life and how I work with clients. It's who I am – authenticity is a key word for me - and I'm helping others also become more authentic too by getting to know their real inner selves. Making the inner connection is key. Becoming more conscious of who they are. Making more conscious choices is all about creating a better life, in harmony with the higher self, Soul and with others and all life around us.

Attaining Good Health Often Requires Change

I am reminded of the expression, if you change nothing, nothing will change. Finding optimum health, I have found, requires a willingness to make changes. Our comfort zones can be very subtle, unnoticeable much of the time. So part of change is really a discovery process - looking at ourselves honestly. This is where contemplation/meditation and other forms of reflection like running, walking, yoga, Pilates and more can be such a great asset helping you to bypass the mental patterns that you have established over the years that may be holding you back now. Also seeing the signs and messages around you can help you get to the heart, to see what needs to shift.

Something Needs to Change

Discovering what needs to shift is the journey. What options or emotional responses to others can you put on the table? How much of your life, the way you go about your life, is open for alteration?

To make changes, you will need to change patterns in your life that are no longer serving your goals and develop new patterns that you need to reach your new goals. My approach is to focus on the things you should start doing: This will allow you to make a shift, leaving the old habits behind. In my experience it will take about a month to establish a new good habit or pattern and personal training can be a great way to establish new patterns in all areas of your life.

By starting with a new exercise routine and making changes to your diet, you can begin the process of finding a new harmony in your life. This can lead to other aspects of your life that also need to shift.

Starting with diet and exercise additions and modifications will in all likelihood change you in ways you had not expected or anticipated. Are you ready for a new you? What is your well-being worth? Is it worth a job, a relationship, giving up assets or things? These are tough questions, but once you are able to let go of certain attachments, discovering the causes and making shifts can be much easier. You may not have to let go of money for example, but by being willing to do so, (for example, letting go of the need for a certain amount of money) opens up new possibilities. This letting go allows us to open up our horizons and allows us to see better choices in our diet, emotional responses, thought patterns and of course, how we keep in shape.

Exercise and diet are a great place to start.

If you don't have the nutrients in your system to recover, much less improve, following intensive exercise, it's like you're flicking a lighter with no butane – you might get a spark but no flame.

Bill Phillips, Body for Life

Four Stages of Exercise

I've found most people fall into one of the following four stages of fitness.

1.   *It's never too late to become what you might have been.* - *George Eliot*

The first stage is a recognition that your health is slipping. You are getting unhealthy and experiencing limitations in your body and as a result in your activities. You recognize that you want to stop this process from getting worse and if possible, reverse the deterioration and regain muscle mass, flexibility and more. I find that a personal fitness consultation can help immeasurably. It will take at least three sessions to get you going on a program designed with your goals in mind.

2.   *The secret of getting ahead is getting started.* - Mark Twain

The second stage is when you decide to take action to reverse the decline. You decide you are not going to be caught up in negative beliefs about aging. After a fitness assessment and some initial training to prevent injury, this is where participation in a small class with more individual attention can help get you turned around and back into good physical condition.

3.   *Strive for progress, not perfection.*

The third stage is a maintenance stage where you settle into a routine of strength training, fitness classes, such as Pilates, yoga etc. and hiking/walking/running. This routine supports your other sports activities such as golf, tennis, cycling and any other sport you choose to round out your fitness maintenance.

4.   *Ability is what you're capable of doing. Motivation determines what you do. Attitude determines how well you do it.* - Lou Holtz

The fourth stage is a specific training program you undertake to participate in a special activity or event like a marathon, triathlon, or charity ride etc. I call this peak performance training to move you beyond your maintenance level to peak physical ability in readiness for your competition. I'm also including in this stage, fitness preparation for a seasonal sport like downhill skiing or golf. This is where personal training can help you get to your very best competitive condition, or slide effortlessly into the next season's sport safely.

The Ideal Routine

It has been proven that the best form of exercise for reshaping your body is strength training (resistance training). Aerobics is excellent, however with strength training you can also increase your fat-burning metabolic rate, so for optimal results a combination of the two is what I recommend. I like to see muscle tissue take up more space than fat tissue. Strength training is even more vital for older adults and one can begin at any age and skill level. An ideal weekly routine is to have a strength training commitment for three days each week and on the alternate days to do something aerobic. Up to twenty minutes of aerobic exercise is enough for most people. (Try burst training.) Exercising longer and more often can be counterproductive. I counsel my clients that low-intensity, long duration aerobic routines (like a long hike) are not as effective at burning fat as a high-intensity workout which boosts the metabolism and keeps it higher for some time following the workout. Having said that, I'm not saying not to go on your hikes or walks...just don't expect a lot of fat-burning from that type of activity.

Another good idea is to work out in the morning in a fasted state (before breakfast) or in a semi-fasted state mid-morning after a light breakfast. This burns fat at a much higher rate than exercise later in the day.

Why Fitness? What Motivates You?

In working with countless clients and students over the years I've found there are several key reasons that motivate people to get in shape and stay in shape thinking holistically - body, emotions, mind and soul. Here are just some of the benefits that may resonate with you:

a) Self Esteem, Self Image: Healthy complexion, improved body shape, muscle definition, better posture, alleviate varicose veins.

b) Disease Prevention: Fitness improves digestion, strengthens the immune system, lowers blood pressure, supports weight loss, improves appetite for healthy foods, strengthens bones, improves liver function.

c) Physical Ability and Enjoyment: Sleep better, have more energy, greater flexibility, strength, endurance, balance, and coordination. Be able to do the things you want to do.

d) Emotional Balance: Self-confidence, emotional stability, foster feelings of well-being, reduce feelings of boredom.

e) Mental Well-being: Relax more quickly, alleviate depression, develop a positive outlook on life, better concentration, let go of annoyances, reduce self-limitations, better problem solving, clearer perspectives on life.

f) Spiritual Harmony: Fitness lifts your spirits, helps you feel good and more alive, opens up new friendships, creates an appreciation for life, helps you attain your fullest potential.

Fitness with Chronic Issues

Many chronic issues are caused by poor food choices. One of the first things I do with clients is to help them see where their current food choices may be causing them problems. As I outlined in my chapter on food choices and environmental toxins, there are many hidden causes of heath issues today. Uncovering these can be as simple as experimentally eliminating a food source such as gluten or high fructose corn syrup for a time to see if that brings about changes for the better.

The second aspect of regaining health while having chronic issues is finding activities that you can participate in, even if you only do a part of a class for example. Simply let the instructor know of your limitations and they'll understand. Or join a special class for people with limitations and chronic conditions. A few personal training sessions can really be a big help in getting started with proper stretching and exercises that work around your issues.

What is Your Perfect Weight?

Does weight really matter? Muscle tissue weighs more than fat but takes up less space, so if you are replacing the space that fat takes up with muscle tissue, know that your weight may not drop, but your pants might! Your weight is primarily influenced by your diet and your exercise.

I don't believe in dieting for the simple reason that it's not sustainable. I've seen clients and students go on extreme regimens, have operations to remove excess skin, only to put all the weight back on a few years later! The best diet is one where you make conscious changes in your food choices that are non-sacrificial. This means substitution of certain foods that are harmful with nutritious foods that taste the same or better. There is no sacrifice involved. It means simply staying with the better choices because you prefer the better choices.

Combining exercise with your diet modifications is the best and most natural way to lose weight and regain a new level of health. One supports the other. Exercise helps your body crave nutrition, and better nutrition helps you exercise more enjoyably.

Optimum Health Weight-loss – My Body-Mind-Soul Permanent Weight Loss Approach

I would be remiss to write a book about health and fitness without talking about my philosophy on weight loss. It seems to be the focus of many people's exercising these days. But achieving weight loss involves so much more than just exercise. I believe for weight loss to work, it needs to address lifestyle changes on all levels as the previous chapters have outlined. The changes I recommend to clients can be very easy for some and more difficult for others. We're all unique! So if you are interested in losing weight and keeping it off, the following four lifestyle modifications are what I include in my client programs.

Weight Loss Lifestyle Modification #1:

Avoid known obesogens, food sources that actually cause obesity.

Obesogens are chemicals, either natural or manmade, that impact the metabolic system, causing one to gain inordinate amounts of weight. Obesogens come from plastics, pesticides and fungicides, soy, chemical sweeteners, and from hormones that are injected into livestock.

It is highly likely you are eating and drinking these chemicals every day. In one study, the obesogen bisphenol-A (BPA) was found in the bodies of 93% of Americans!

Obesogens are thought to affect us by interfering with the regulatory systems that control body weight. That's why following traditional advice won't lower your obesogen exposure.

Here are some tips...

Cut Down Your Pesticide/Chemicals Exposure

The average North American is exposed to about 13 different pesticides through food, beverages and drinking water every day, and 9 of the 10 most common pesticides are obesogens. Eating an organic diet can reduce unwanted chemicals in your body to non-detectable levels.

Of course, organic foods can be expensive. But not all organics are created equal – many foods have such low levels of pesticides that buying organic may not be worth it for you. You can reduce your pesticide exposure nearly 80% simply by choosing organic for the 12 fruits and vegetables shown in tests to contain the highest levels of pesticides which some call the dirty dozen:

I recommend focussing on organically grown versions of these foods - the worst are on the top of this list:

- Peaches
- Apples
- Sweet Bell Peppers
- Celery
- Nectarines
- Strawberries
- Cherries
- Kale
- Lettuce
- Imported Grapes
- Carrots
- Pears

The following have been shown to have little pesticide residue, so conventionally grown versions of these foods are reported to be fine.

- Onions
- Avocados
- Sweet Corn (avoid if genetically modified)
- Pineapples
- Mangoes
- Asparagus
- Sweet Peas
- Kiwis
- Cabbages
- Eggplants
- Papayas
- Watermelons
- Broccoli
- Tomatoes
- Sweet Potatoes

A Seafood Cautionary

By the way, avoiding pesticides means choosing seafood wisely, as well. For example, Atlantic salmon (all of which is farm-raised) has up to 90% more pesticides than wild-caught Alaskan/Pacific salmon.

Don't Drink or Eat From Plastic

Phthalates, another obesogen are synthetic chemicals found in plastics that lower testosterone, and trick our bodies into storing fat. Here's what you can do to reduce your exposure:

1. Never heat food in plastic containers or put plastic items such as water bottles in the dishwasher, which can damage them and increase leaching.

2. As mentioned in chapter 2, avoid buying fatty foods like meats that are packaged in plastic wrap. Plastic wrap used in

supermarkets is mostly PVC, a type of plastic that leaches phthalates; like other obesogens, phthalates are attracted to, and are stored in, fatty tissue. Alternatively, ask the meat department staff to wrap your meat in paper. (Don't worry about Saran Wrap or other plastic wrap as most are made from polyethylene, a less troublesome type of plastic.)

3. Cut down on canned goods by choosing fresh or frozen vegetables or tuna in a pouch over canned tuna.

Organic Free Range Beef

If you eat beef, choose organic, pasture-raised meats whenever possible, for two reasons: First, avoiding obesogens is all about protecting your hormonal system. But conventionally raised beef comes preloaded with six different hormones including the weight-gain hormone TBA; those hormones are used to make the cows gain weight, and they're still detectable in the meat after slaughter. Second, grass-fed beef is leaner, contains 60% more omega-3s, 200% more vitamin E and 2-3 times more conjugated linoleic acid (a near-magic nutrient that helps ward off heart disease, cancer and diabetes, and can help you lose weight) than conventional beef.

Filter Your Water

The best way to eliminate obesogens from your water is an activated carbon water filter.

Fast Food/Junk Food

Avoid fast foods and junk foods: they usually contain multiple obesogens such as sugar, sugar substitutes and high fructose corn syrup, oils that are rancid, preservatives and other suspect ingredients.

Mainstream/chain restaurants are no better; many of their dishes are factory made, frozen, then reheated for you. Eat organic if possible when dining out or select proprietor-owned restaurants where they take pride in their ingredients and will cater to you substitutions, your more conscious choices!

Weight Loss Lifestyle Modification #2:

Align your food choices with your weight loss goals.

Review chapter two and follow these recommendations:

Eliminate North American wheat

Eliminate sugar and chemical sugar substitutes

Eliminate rancid oils

Avoid processed foods

Weight Loss Lifestyle Modification #3:

Be open to self-examination

Emotions, thoughts and beliefs that are part of your life lesson plan may need modification/purification.

Be willing to uncover deeply seeded patterns from your past that could be within your genetic make-up (predispositions). Open yourself to changing your core beliefs.

No diet will ever be successful if you don't go to that place inside you, a place usually wrapped in pain, discomfort, shame, self-defeating habits, and fear. Unless you take care of this inner place, this inner fat person who is hiding from the world and herself or himself, then no matter what the diet, it will not work in the long run.

Tosco Reno, The Start Here Diet

Weight Loss Lifestyle Modification #4:

Adopt a regular comprehensive fitness and sports lifestyle that is enjoyable for you.

Getting Fit is Simple...But Not Necessarily Easy!

Decide what you want to achieve. From the list of spiritual qualities of health and harmony at the back of this book, make a note of the key areas that motivate you. Circle five.

Schedule the time. Are you a morning, mid-day, afternoon or evening person? (Morning workouts on an empty stomach are best for fat loss.)

Start with modest goals. Don't make it too hard. Get a trainer to assist you with your new direction.

Create variety by mixing sports with fitness classes or personal workouts. Balance is important.

Have a dedicated place for your fitness activities (home gym, fitness club, sports location)

Be the best you can be!

Setting Goals

I like to say that a goal is a self-promise. You need to pledge to yourself that your commitments are sacred. I believe keeping one's fitness vows unleashes great potential and energy and results in feelings of accomplishment. This has the effect of translating into higher self-esteem and confidence in life. Find a way to give yourself an incentive (not a big dinner out, by-the-way!) For many, it's entering a charity competition. For others it is having something at stake, anything to create the drive to reach one's goals like a special trip as a reward for your hard work and achievements.

A "spiritual" tip in creating successful change is to work with the spiritual principle of reflection. It involves taking your attention off yourself and focussing on others. Think about others in your circle of family and friends that you can support in some way. Think of ways to compliment them or do something positive for them. You could even do this without them knowing – a silent act of love. Look for the good in others and speak only positively of others and your outlook will change: It will be a reflection of what you are projecting to others. You will move into a new positive world that you have created. We can actually re-create our world and our future this way.

What You Should Expect from Personal Training

Sometimes, a little help and motivation go a long way on the road to overall fitness. Studies show you can achieve you goals three times faster than exercising on your own. You should expect to receive personalized programming for your body type and for your goals, limitations and needs. This will maximize your time in your workouts. With your trainer, you should learn safety and injury prevention working with equipment or without for example in running, stretching etc. You should be offered a variety of types of training to keep your program fresh and motivating and you should also receive a progression of exercises in your routine to keep you improving. Most important, your trainer should be genuinely interested in you and your lifestyle, not simply be a "fitness baby sitter" or a "workout buddy."

A Holistic Approach

My mission is to offer a holistic service that helps my clients reach their full potential for health, happiness and balance in their life. In addition I want to be there for my clients with their challenges and help them break new ground in achieving their dreams and goals.

Your goals come from your dreams. Powerful dreams of positive changes in your life add even more fuel to your transformation. But you must create goals that are in sync with your dreams in order to move forward in your life and feel good about yourself, your progress, and your future potential.

Bill Phillips, author of Body for Life

I assist clients on several levels, a complete Body-Mind-Soul approach - (physical, emotional, mental and spiritual), depending on what their needs are. Clients can access, if they choose, the following elements which are integral to my personal training services:

1) Fitness (physical) training that can include:

Structural yoga therapy, Pilates, strength training, and chakra (energy) balancing technique sessions. These can be combined with several other fitness disciplines to engage/challenge each client at their specific level - based on their personal capabilities, limitations, or injuries.

2) Essential oil aromatherapy when appropriate.

Aromatherapy is the therapeutic use of essential oils, highly aromatic substances that naturally occur in plants. It combines chemistry, biology, and botany with intuition in the blending of various oils that create therapeutic or beneficial effects. Many of my blends offer a tangible and powerful aid to physical and emotional healing and lifestyle and anti-aging issues. Others provide natural alternatives to household chemical cleaners.

3) I am also able to engage clients on a spiritual level if they choose, understanding each individual's unique life-experience. In this area of service I utilize my 16 years of spiritual study to enhance a client's sense of well-being and lifestyle. This may include the use of contemplation practices.

4) Massage and Reflexology Treatments.

I offer three key services to help clients rebalance, rejuvenate and de-stress:

Aromatherapy Massage is a relaxing, healing and soothing massage with a custom blend of pure essential oils helps to stimulate circulation and induce relaxation.

Reflexology - This ancient holistic and healing therapy is designed to restore the body to a healthy balance. A combination of massage techniques and pressure point work is performed on the feet to help create a sense of inner calm and rejuvenation.

Ocean Stone Massage is a favorite among clients - smooth, heated basalt stones and chilled marble stones work their way into tired and stressed tissue leaving you feeling in seventh heaven. The ultimate relaxation of body, mind and soul.

5) Dietary evaluation and ongoing guidance on important health considerations including, if requested a pantry/cupboard evaluation in the home.

How I Work with Clients

I only work with clients whose goals I can support with enthusiasm and who are prepared to commit to their better health and fitness.

Through tailored exercise programs, I enjoy helping people from all walks of life and with all kinds of limitations to meet their fitness and health goals. The overall goal of my training programs is to assist clients in achieving physical fitness benefits effectively in combination with healthy lifestyle and nutritional advice.

To achieve this goal, I set the following objectives:

1. Clear and realistic physical fitness goals that are customized to a client's specific needs and challenges as follows:

   How fitness goals will be achieved;
   Amount of work needed to reach goals;
   Types of activities desired to reach goals; Frequency and intensity of workouts;

2. Recommend and instruct on proper exercise techniques.

   I teach safe and effective use of equipment to avoid injury;
   Proper body mechanics; and I
   Develop and provide customized exercises that suit your individual fitness needs.

3. Individualize a physical fitness workout program:

I incorporate the components of total fitness including muscular endurance, muscular strength, flexibility, and cardiovascular conditioning;
Personally guide each fitness workout;
Monitor progress and adjust workouts accordingly;
Provide accountability and motivation in achieving fitness goals.

4. Provide cutting edge information and guidance in training and nutrition:
I study extensively and subscribe to the latest fitness, health, yoga, Pilates, personal training and heath books and journals, and attend world-class fitness conferences, incorporating state-of-the-art thinking and research into all of my client programs.

My Body-Mind-Soul (Holistic) Fitness Philosophy

The following points are a brief synopsis of my beliefs for maintaining excellent health:

1. Good Health is dependent on harmony of your total being: a balance of body, emotions, mind and soul.

2. Exercise is vital for health and longevity.

3. Exercise also supports our learning processes.

4. We also need rest. Get lots.

5. Drink at least 2 litres of water each day.

7. Over exercising can cause health issues.

8. Love your body. What you do with it affects your whole self.

9. Have fun! Movement and play go hand-in-hand.

10. Laugh a lot. Give joy to others. Get outside and be with nature.

11. Eat the cleanest foods you can.

12. Know that setbacks are a part of life; it seems it is when we are really tested that we grow the most. So recognize that you are bound to experience adversity and try to see it as a springboard to a greater consciousness, a higher perspective of greater self-confidence and self-trust. Others often hear me say, "build a bridge and get over it."

Fit is not a destination, it's a way of life!

Final Thoughts

Think of your body as a finely tuned machine. You have to feed it the right fuel, the best fuel, and you have to take care of the engine and give it regular fine-tunings. This is just common sense. You will be the recipient of negative consequences if you put into your body chemicals and bad oils (that is, trans fats, hydrogenated oils, artificial food, and poison), if you don't sleep properly and long enough, or if you load up with pharmaceuticals without thought about the effect they are having. If you don't think good thoughts, if you wallow in negatives, what do you think will manifest?

We are what we eat, think, and drink.

Suzanne Somers, Ageless

It Really Comes Down to Making More Conscious Choices

The main theme of this book has been about making more conscious choices — and when you are willing to open in this way, new realizations about yourself can flood in, bringing a rebalancing and harmony at all levels. I invite you to move forward on your life-journey into excellent well-being by thinking about the choices you are making in foods, your environment and emotional responses. I encourage you to become more aware of how your thoughts are shaping your present and future and to spend time each day in contemplation, a time just for you.

Making conscious choices in all of these areas of your life is the key to good health and enthusiasm for life!

Ultimately, you are the only one who can make significant deposits into your health bank account. This is not the job of your doctor, nutritionist, your lover or your parents. There is no supplement, no health care provider, and no exotic herb that can possibly do for you what you can do for yourself.

Cristiane Northrup, MD, The Wisdom of Menopause

Appendix

Spiritual Qualities for Health and Harmony

Honesty, Forgiveness, Humor, Love, Detachment, Contentment, Humility, Joy, Enthusiasm, Sharing, Respect, Flexibility, Trust, Harmony, Listening, Caring, Empathy, Grace, Charity, Discipline, Order, Purity, Kindness, Freedom, Openness, Truthfulness, Nurturing, Loyalty, Ingenuity, Discretion, Effectiveness, Reliability, Resourcefulness, Service, Clarity, Prosperity, Commitment, Punctuality, Neatness, Excellence, Optimism, Accuracy, Achievement, Originality, Admiration, Organization, Advancement, Persistence, Personal Growth, Appreciation, Frankness, Friendship, Education, Efficiency, Encouragement, Mastery, Fun, Volunteerism, Cooperation, Acceptance, Gratitude, Thankfulness, Openness, Helpfulness, Cheerfulness, Responsibility, Serenity, Communication, Inspiration, Abundance, Beauty, Play, Compassion, Strength, Surrender, Tenderness, Adventure, Faith, Peace, Balance, Patience, Flexibility, Transformation, Courage, Release, Spontaneity, Integrity, Willingness, Healing, Right Discrimination (making right choices), Simplicity, Purpose, Synthesis, Confident, Enthusiastic, Faithful, Happy, Positive, Sincerity, Tolerant, Understanding, Courage, Supportive, Giving, Hopeful

These qualities are aspects of love!

About the Author

Andrea Switzer has integrated many enlightened practices into her daily life and as a health and fitness leader she walks her talk: Her personal body-mind-soul philosophy is her foundation in life. "This set of personal values helps me weather the storms of change, setbacks and unexpected outcomes, whether it be physically, emotionally, mentally or spiritually," she tells others. She loves to pass along her holistic insights to her clients, students, family and friends.

Andrea combines over 20 years of passion for health and fitness with a love for providing service excellence in all she does. As a teacher, coach, and trainer she also considers herself to be a life-long student, bringing to her clients state-of-the-art practices from health and fitness seminars, conferences, video presentations, books and journals. She recognizes the divine spark in everyone and she is also one to recognize the value in learning from those she connects with as well.

A graduate of Simon Fraser University, Andrea studied kinesiology, anatomy, nutrition, physiology, and fitness programming. She has taken numerous courses and certifications, constantly upgrading her skills, and is certified in 'The Method' Pilates (Physicalmind Institute) and in Yoga (East West Yoga, Toronto, Ontario).

She has provided personal fitness training to discerning and high-profile clients for fifteen years, offering highly customized client training using many fitness disciplines ranging from Pilates and Yoga, TRX Suspension Training, Gravity Training, concurrently with many other strength training modalities, as well as post-training flexibility techniques. She has been a certified fitness leader for over 20 years and was Assistant Director at Canada's largest YMCA in Toronto, responsible for fitness program delivery.

Andrea has also enjoyed working with clients with physical mobility challenges and degenerative issues to help them maintain and recover their lifestyles. She has been teaching mind/body disciplines (Yoga and Pilates) for all levels for over 15 years, helping individuals achieve a new balance and a renewed sense of well-being in their lives.

She is also certified through the Holt School of Natural Healing, Caledon, Ontario as an Aromatherapist and as well, is certified in Hot/Cold Stone Massage Therapy by Ocean Stone Therapy, Vancouver, British Columbia. Andrea was spa director at Upper Mission Spa, and also worked as a spa therapist and continues to provide relaxation massage services and Reflexology for private clients.

Optimum Health: Making Conscious Choices, encompasses much of what is Andrea – the disciplined practice of daily contemplation, yoga and Pilates for balance and physical exercise and a constant assessment of the latest health and fitness thinking and practices that is as much for her enjoyment and relaxation as for passing along to her students and clients.